Wall Pilates 101

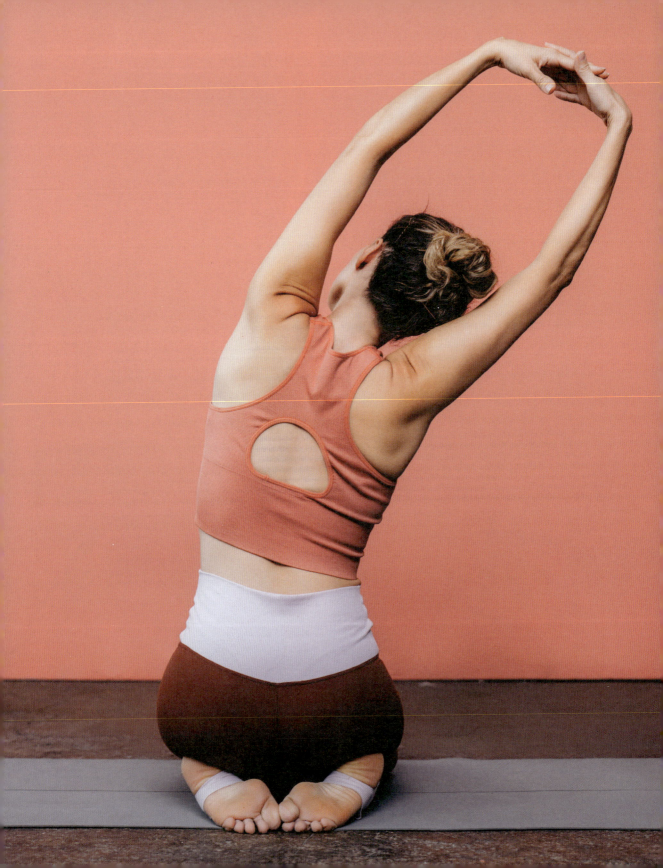

Prevention

Wall Pilates 101

THE LOW-IMPACT WAY TO BOOST FLEXIBILITY BUILD BALANCE & LOOK FIT

KATHRYN ROSS-NASH & THE EDITORS OF PREVENTION

TABLE OF CONTENTS

Exercise Glossary
WARMUP EXERCISES

COOLDOWN EXERCISES

WORKOUT EXERCISES

STANDING EXERCISES

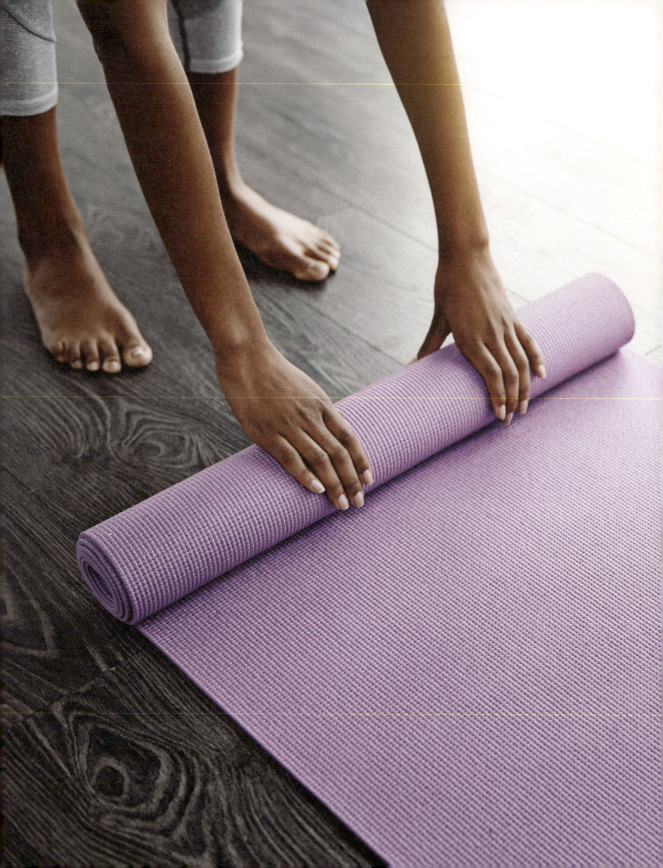

Pilates for Real Life

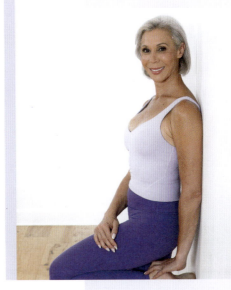

Some fitness activities seem impossible to work into everyday life. Training for an ultramarathon or taking up CrossFit, for example, requires lots of time and energy, a combo that can be hard to come by for most of us. And another such activity—at least at first glance—is Pilates. This workout system typically involves specialized equipment that you can access either at a Pilates studio or, if you're willing to shell out hundreds of dollars, in your home gym. So if you don't live near a studio or can't get your own equipment, Pilates might not seem like the kind of fitness regimen you can engage in regularly.

I used to feel the same way. In 1982, I was a principal dancer in need of an exercise program that could lengthen my muscles and help me avoid injuries in the dance studio. I took weekly Pilates classes with my mentor and teacher, Romana Kryzanowska, and the work we did was transformative. I felt flexible, light on my feet, and strong. I wanted to practice beyond our weekly meetups—but at home, without the benefit of a studio full of equipment, I wasn't sure it'd be the same. I tried hooking my feet under the sofa and exercising on my bed, a yoga mat, and the carpet. Nothing felt quite right.

I started to worry that my goal of doing Pilates at home would prove unattainable. But then I remembered how Romana and I ended so many of our Pilates sessions: Against the wall! A wall was definitely something I had access to, so I tried using it for my at-home Pilates workouts. It gave me just what I was looking for. I could replicate the constraints of the equipment and of Romana's hands, and give myself the precise amount of resistance I needed.

Since then, I've continued to use a wall as part of my Pilates practice and the routines I create for clients. While I was traveling for 10 years as a professional ballerina, I relied on walls in hotel rooms for workouts, rather than trying to get to a local Pilates studio. When I create workout programs for people looking to improve their strength, mobility, and flexibility, I always include wall work. I've seen it help countless clients maintain their practice even with busy schedules and travel, paving the way for long-term wellness. If you're looking to start doing Pilates, there's no better place to begin than the wall.

Over the years I've learned the best exercises to recreate all the amazing benefits of a Pilates workout—strength, flexibility, and toned arms, legs, and abs—using nothing but a wall. And now I want to share those secrets with you. In this book you'll find my four-week plan featuring the exact exercises you need to build long, lean muscles, just like the results you'd get from regular sessions in a Pilates studio. Each exercise will stretch, strengthen, and tone your muscles, center your mind, and bring balance to both. You'll safely explore new exercises without having to navigate unfamiliar equipment, and you'll do it all from the comfort of your home.

Even today, with a studio full of every type of Pilates equipment imaginable, I teach wall Pilates at every level to clients, students, and teachers. With the wall exercises in this book, you'll build the strength and flexibility needed to better support your muscles from head to toe. That will help you build more power to move through your day, maintain better balance during your daily activities, and refine your motor skills. Rest assured, you'll never look at a simple wall in quite the same way again.

KATHRYN ROSS-NASH

Wall Pilates 101

What Is Wall Pilates?

Step into any Pilates studio and you'll see lots of specialized equipment, such as bands, rings, and large machines such as the Reformer and chair. Those things can give you a great workout. But if you want to keep it simple while still getting big results, all you really need is a wall.

If you're new to Pilates, let's start with the basics. The traditional Pilates method is a form of strength training that improves muscle tone, core strength, and flexibility while boosting your endurance and stability. But unlike other resistance exercises such as weight training, it utilizes small, controlled movements to give users long, lean muscles. (In fact, Pilates was developed as a way

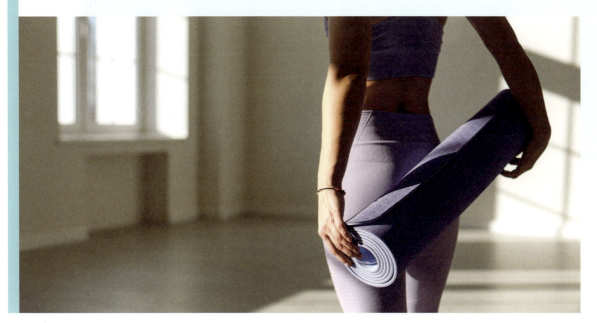

for ballerinas to stay in shape!) What's more, Pilates is low impact so it's gentle on your joints. It's ideal for anyone looking to get stronger and more toned without high-intensity exercises or heavy weights.

Wall Pilates does the same exact things as traditional Pilates, only without the expensive equipment. Instead of using a Reformer or another device for resistance, the resistance comes simply from pressing your hands, feet, back, or other body part against a wall while performing the exercises. You'll get some extra support and stability when you need it too, like with inversion exercises where your feet are above your head as you lie on the ground. Basically, it gives you all the good stuff without any equipment. If you're wondering how that's possible, read on for more on how wall Pilates mimics the effects of its traditional counterpart.

KEEPS YOUR FORM
IN CHECK

You know the saying "quality over quantity"? That concept is critical when it comes to seeing results from your workouts. Ensuring that your body is in the correct position for every exercise is especially important in Pilates, where every movement is small but precise. Performing moves with your body improperly aligned can negate its benefits, or worse, result in injury.

In a Pilates studio, you'd have a combination of teachers and tools to correct your form. You'd use the Reformer (a device that looks like a bed frame with ropes, pulleys, and springs) to help you find proper alignment, as well as to provide resistance to push against. To feel if your weight is equally distributed across your pelvis, ribs, and shoulders, you would press your back against the carriage bed, or base of the tool. To do the same for your hands, you would place them on the foot bar and shoulder blocks. And for your feet, you'd use the foot bar.

In wall Pilates, you simply use the wall to find all those points of pressure, contact, and balance, and also to ascertain that you're performing an exercise correctly. Throughout this plan, you'll perform moves that situate your feet, back, or the side of your body on the wall, allowing you to check your form and get the most from every exercise. Plus, you'll get detailed, step-by-step directions for every move in this program so you can always be sure you're acing your technique.

ADAPTS
TO ALL FITNESS LEVELS

In order for your muscles to get toned, they have to be met with some type of resistance. Depending on the workout you do, that resistance might come in the form of dumbbells, resistance

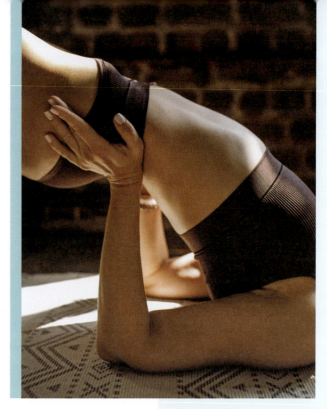

bands, or your own body weight. During a traditional Pilates session, that resistance typically comes from the Reformer. The Reformer has springs that determine the level of resistance you'll encounter as you do an exercise. You might do moves that require pushing or pulling on those springs, all of which help create lean, toned muscle. However, the springs on the Reformer have fixed tensions, meaning you have little control over the intensity of your workout.

Wall Pilates allows for more customization. At home, you get to decide how much resistance you want, based on the amount of pressure you place against the wall, with little to no impact on your joints. It's all in the way you position your body. Imagine trying to do a push-up with your hands on a wall. If you stand very close to the wall so your body is nearly parallel to it, the push-up will be easier. If you stand farther back so your body is at a 45-degree angle to the wall, it will be harder. You'll get this same flexibility with the plan in this book. Plus, with no moving parts involved, you'll have less to think about, which means you can zero in on what feels right.

PROVIDES
STABILITY

When you're struggling to maintain your balance, it's hard to get any benefit from an exercise. For example, the lunge is a great exercise for toning your lower body, but if you're wobbling your way through lunges, they won't do much for you.

For some people, finding balance while on the Reformer in a traditional Pilates setting is challenging. Taking your practice to the wall means you have a stable place to lean. The wall offers support when you lose your footing and also allows you to safely test the limits of your balance. End result? You can focus more of your attention on activating the muscles you want to tone.

The wall is your safety net. You can lean on it, push onto it, and peel off of it with ease. It can help you perform exercises that you might not yet have the balance or strength to do without it. For example, the hundred (page 88) is a highly effective exercise for sculpting your abs, but it can be difficult for beginners. When you utilize a wall as

a place to rest your feet, you alleviate some of the challenging elements while still firing up your core.

The stability you'll get from the wall also allows you to direct more of your attention toward the parts of your body that you're not moving. That's right—I said not moving. Many exercises focus on keeping certain body parts in motion, like lifting your feet when you walk or raising a dumbbell for an overhead press. In a Pilates wall workout, you'll build strength and stamina by paying equal attention to what's staying still.

Take the double-leg stretch on page 104, for example. Your feet are placed on the wall, and they don't move. But as you roll your pelvis off the mat and lift your ankles and knees, the pressure on your feet increases. Keeping them steady on the wall takes a lot of effort! This effort builds strength and mobility in the deeper, stabilizing muscles throughout your lower body.

The hundred is another example of this. You pump your arms vigorously while performing the move, but the hardest work is not allowing your legs or torso to move. If you pump your arms and let your legs or torso move, you won't get the same muscle-toning benefits and could even end up hurting your back. Don't be afraid to use the wall for support—that's what it's there for!

WHY YOU'LL LOVE WALL PILATES

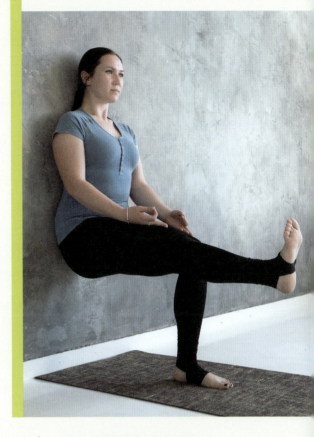

It's clear that wall Pilates translates some of the most important elements of traditional Pilates into easy at-home exercises. Now let's learn what makes this workout so fantastic and how these simple moves can make you stronger, healthier, and leaner. Here are just some of the things a regular wall Pilates practice can do.

IT SAVES YOU TIME

A well-rounded exercise program should include resistance exercises, cardiovascular exercises, and stretching and flexibility exercises. Many workouts hit just one of these points; lifting a weight is a resistance move, for example, while jogging is strictly cardio. With wall Pilates, you get all three at the same time: You work and stretch your muscles while elevating your heart rate to burn calories. It's a powerful combo for sculpting long, lean muscle. In short, you get the biggest workout bang for your buck.

IT TONES YOUR WHOLE BODY

You don't need a rack of dumbbells or even a gym membership to tone up from head to toe. In order to sculpt your arms, abs, legs, and glutes, you just need to challenge them with a resisting force. In wall Pilates, those resisting forces are gravity and a wall. You'll perform small, repeated movements with one body part while isolating other body parts to carve lean, powerful muscles without bulking up.

What's more, you won't spend precious time focusing on individual muscles, like your biceps or triceps. While each exercise has a specific target area (like the legs, arms, or abs), you'll find that you need to activate *all* of your muscles to remain stable. As a result, every part of your body is challenged—and gets stronger.

IT FEELS GOOD

You may think Pilates is primarily used to strengthen and tone your body, but in many of the exercises you'll also get a good stretch. You'll bend and twist and reach for your toes while also sculpting lean muscle. A 2015 study found that people who practiced Pilates just three times a week showed increased hamstring flexibility—which is especially important to avoid injury from walking or running. Better flexibility can reduce your risk of injury in general by relieving stiff muscles, thereby allowing you to move with more control. An added bonus: Stretching can lower your stress levels.

IT SUPPORTS WEIGHT LOSS

The resistance work you'll do during your Pilates wall workouts will not only tone your muscles but also help you build *more* muscle—without the need for lifting weights. And that can translate to pounds lost. You'll feel slimmer and more comfortable in your clothes, since a regular Pilates practice delivers long, lean muscles, not big or bulky ones.

That's because your body uses more energy to maintain muscle tissue than it does fat. So when you build muscle, your body torches more calories throughout the day even when you're not exercising. (Talk about a return on your investment.) The upshot? You get closer to your weight loss goals.

IT MAKES
EVERYDAY TASKS EASIER

From the moment you step out of bed in the morning to when you brush your teeth at night, your daily life requires you to perform a huge range of motions. You twist your torso in the car to check your blind spot, bend your legs to plug in your laptop, and raise your arms to grab plates off a high shelf. The strengthening, balancing, and breathing exercises in your Pilates wall workouts will engage your muscles in the same ways. That means you'll be better equipped to perform everyday movements and tasks with a little more ease.

IT REDUCES INJURY RISK

Nothing derails a fitness goal like getting sidelined by an injury. And more often than not, workout-related mishaps, like muscle pulls or strains, often stem from simply doing too much too soon.

Like all Pilates workouts, the workouts in this plan build gradually to prepare your body for what's next. In each workout, you'll ease into things with the gentlest moves and slowly kick up the intensity, all while focusing on proper form. That way there's less risk of pushing yourself too far too quickly. You'll also curb the kind of muscle tension that can make you tight or uncomfortable, since wall Pilates includes plenty of feel-good stretching. And since the moves in this program are low-impact, you'll always be going easy on your joints.

And let's not forget that the strong, sturdy core you'll build from wall Pilates can help you avert all kinds of injuries. If you trip over floor clutter or slip on an icy walkway, for instance, a stable midsection makes regaining your balance much easier. You'll be less prone to falls as you go about your day.

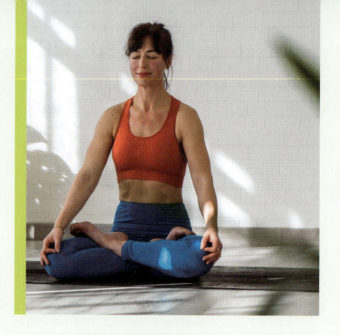

IT CAN BOOST
YOUR MOOD

The exercises in this book will benefit not only your body but also your mind. Physical activity is a proven stress reliever and mood booster, and that's especially true of wall Pilates. Deep belly breaths, which you'll take while performing the moves in this plan, trigger physiological responses that have a near-instant calming effect.

You may reap cognitive benefits too. The exercises that involve crossing your midline (like the spine twist on page 128) signal communication between the two sides of your brain. This spurs the development of new neural pathways that support emotional resilience as well as critical thinking and problem solving. The inversions (like the lying with legs up the wall exercise on page 135) are known to be superchargers for your brain; they can also help regulate blood pressure, aid digestion, and calm your mind.

IT CAN BE DONE
(ALMOST) ANYWHERE

Unlike traditional Pilates, wall Pilates can be done wherever there's a wall, making it ultra-convenient. If you're short on time or feeling unmotivated, you don't have to travel far to start your workout; that means you'll be more likely to stick to a regular practice. Whether you're at home or away, it's usually pretty easy to find some empty wall space where you can work out. And if you can't, just move the furniture!

Who Is Wall Pilates For?

LET'S FACE IT: Starting an exercise program like Pilates can be intimidating. It's enough to make you wonder if Pilates is the right fit for you. Luckily, this wall Pilates plan takes the guesswork out of every exercise, making it approachable to almost anyone. If you fall into any of the following categories, this program is for you!

Newcomers to Pilates

Wall workouts are my go-to for beginners. Learning new exercises while navigating an unfamiliar piece of equipment, like a Reformer, can be overwhelming. When you take the extra equipment out of the equation and just use a wall, you can focus solely on mastering the movements. And there's no need to commit to a gym or a studio or buy expensive gear. If you commit to wall Pilates, I promise you'll see—and feel!—real results.

People with Limited Mobility

Wall Pilates is also a great choice if you have limited mobility, because the wall is a stable and supportive partner. If you're able to lower yourself to the floor and lift yourself back up, you'll be able to succeed with this workout. You might even find that a regular wall Pilates practice improves your mobility over time, by boosting your flexibility or helping to relieve problems like chronic back pain.

Anyone Looking for a Convenient, Effective Full-Body Workout

Traditional Pilates builds balanced muscle development with controlled, functional movements while giving you a great stretch. It tests your balance too, so you're steadier on your feet for everyday movements like walking, running, or going up and down stairs. Wall Pilates does the same exact thing, in a way that's more approachable. You'll work your body from head to toe—all with nothing but a wall!

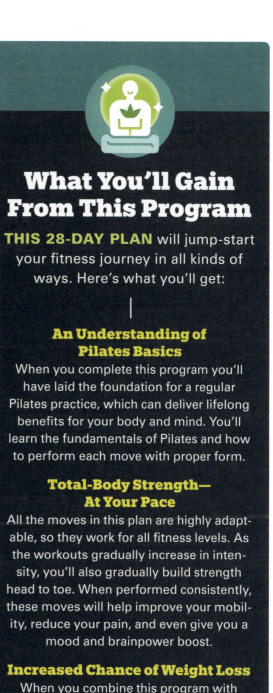

What You'll Gain From This Program

THIS 28-DAY PLAN will jump-start your fitness journey in all kinds of ways. Here's what you'll get:

An Understanding of Pilates Basics

When you complete this program you'll have laid the foundation for a regular Pilates practice, which can deliver lifelong benefits for your body and mind. You'll learn the fundamentals of Pilates and how to perform each move with proper form.

Total-Body Strength— At Your Pace

All the moves in this plan are highly adaptable, so they work for all fitness levels. As the workouts gradually increase in intensity, you'll also gradually build strength head to toe. When performed consistently, these moves will help improve your mobility, reduce your pain, and even give you a mood and brainpower boost.

Increased Chance of Weight Loss

When you combine this program with a healthy balanced diet, you'll find that your clothes fit more comfortably and you might even lose a pound or two. All that from some simple wall exercises!

The Secret to Getting Real Results

YOU MIGHT BE TEMPTED to jump right to the 28-day plan, but if you spend a few minutes absorbing the helpful hints in this chapter, your wall Pilates journey will be all the better for it. When starting any new routine, it's normal to run into obstacles that threaten your results. You may have trouble mastering a move, or you may have days when you don't feel like working out at all. The tips I'll share with you here have helped my clients (and myself!) see real progress in their Pilates practice, and I know they'll work for you too.

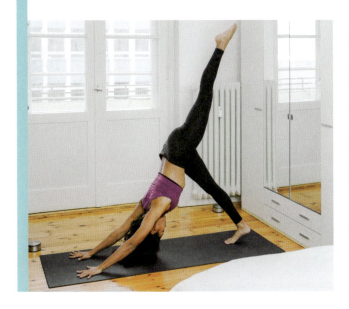

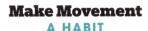

Make Movement
A HABIT

When you perform a task regularly, such as brushing your teeth in the morning, it eventually becomes second nature. Exercise can be the same. Try to make a point of getting some form of physical activity every day. On the days when you don't work out, use that time to move your body in another way. Go for a walk or do some stretching. I know this sounds a little daunting! But you really will reap the biggest benefits by committing to daily movement, even if it's just for a half hour. (That's about how long each Pilates workout is.)

Think of it this way: Daily exercise is a gift you give to yourself. I'm sure if a loved one asked you to spare 30 minutes a day to make *their* lives better, you'd make time for them. Don't you deserve the same for yourself? We commit to everyone else; now it's time to commit to you.

Use
YOUR WHOLE BODY

Each exercise in this program targets a specific area of the body, like the abs, arms, or legs. But you can—and should!—try to engage your entire body as you perform each move. When you utilize as many muscles as possible, you'll get more

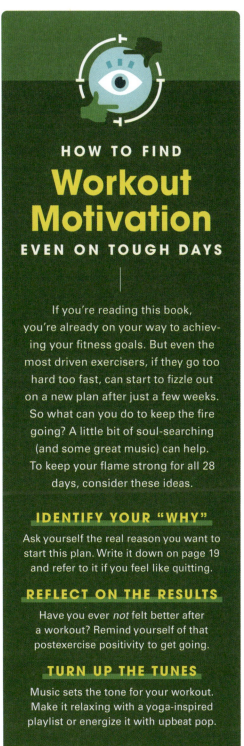

HOW TO FIND
Workout Motivation
EVEN ON TOUGH DAYS

If you're reading this book, you're already on your way to achieving your fitness goals. But even the most driven exercisers, if they go too hard too fast, can start to fizzle out on a new plan after just a few weeks. So what can you do to keep the fire going? A little bit of soul-searching (and some great music) can help. To keep your flame strong for all 28 days, consider these ideas.

IDENTIFY YOUR "WHY"
Ask yourself the real reason you want to start this plan. Write it down on page 19 and refer to it if you feel like quitting.

REFLECT ON THE RESULTS
Have you ever *not* felt better after a workout? Remind yourself of that postexercise positivity to get going.

TURN UP THE TUNES
Music sets the tone for your workout. Make it relaxing with a yoga-inspired playlist or energize it with upbeat pop.

strength-building, calorie-burning bang for your buck and come closer to seeing results faster. Full-body awareness also helps you maintain better alignment, which reduces your risk for potential injuries.

Take the cross-leg twist (page 85), for example. In addition to focusing on lifting your upper body and bicycling your legs, pay attention to the part of your body that's not moving: your core. This area stays anchored throughout the exercise, giving you a stabilizing place from which to move and stretch.

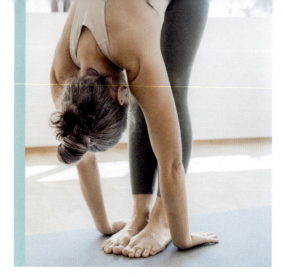

Fine-Tune
YOUR FORM

As I mentioned, wall Pilates is all about quality over quantity, so try to do each move as prescribed. You'll reap more benefits from an exercise by doing a handful of strong, well-aligned repetitions than by cranking out tons of so-so ones.

If you're new to Pilates, I recommend reading the directions for each exercise three times to get a feel for it before your workout. Also, check out the photos to get a visual for what the exercise looks like. Sure, the exercise still might feel a little wobbly the first couple of times you do it. Just try your best to follow the instructions! After a few workouts, the moves will start to feel more natural and you won't have to keep peeking at the directions.

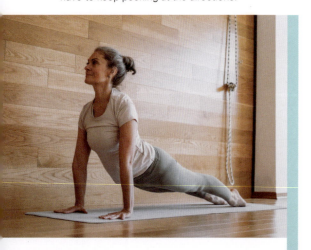

Keeping tabs on your form gives you more than just a better Pilates workout, by the way. Maintaining proper alignment while you exercise will help you maintain better alignment in your everyday life. Bearing more weight on one hip when you're standing or walking, for instance, can cause extra wear and tear on that hip and result in pain and inflammation. The side-kick series exercise (page 124) will help you strengthen both hips equally, making you less prone to leaning to one side throughout the day. Do you play a one-sided sport like golf and are always swinging in one direction? You'll love the spine twist exercise (page 128), which can improve your rotational balance and help you swing more evenly.

Warm Up
AND COOL DOWN

Each workout in this plan includes a warmup and a cooldown. Even if you're feeling rushed, don't skip them! Taking the extra few minutes is always worth it. Your warmup prepares your body for the stress of exercise by bringing more blood to your muscles, helping you loosen up and reduce your risk for injury. And your cooldown gradually lowers your heart rate, allowing your body to gently return to a state of rest.

You can use the warmup or cooldown as their own mini-workouts too. A round of the hug with elbow lift exercise (page 134) can release some tension and rev you up before you go on to tackle the rest of your day. A few minutes spent on the lying with legs up the wall exercise (page 135), on the other hand, can help you unwind and find your center after a hard day.

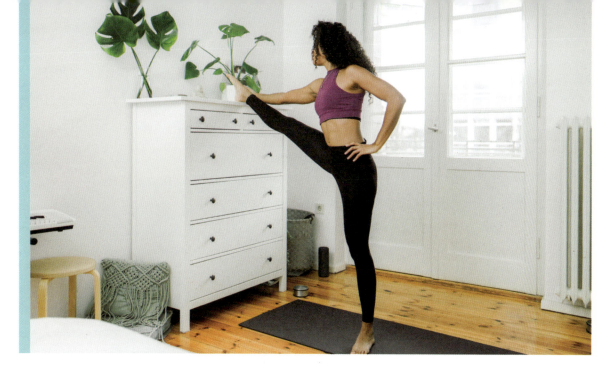

Bring Your Mind
TO THE MAT

In Pilates class, we like to say, "Try not to think about what you've done in the past or anticipate how you think an exercise should feel. Rather, experience it as you execute it."

Put another way? Stay in the moment while you practice; see how it makes you feel, and respond accordingly. In all of these wall Pilates moves, a part of your body will be in contact with the wall, and a part of your body will be in contact with the floor. Pay attention to both of them. Then notice what happens when you move. Where do you feel the deepest stretch? How does your weight shift? Keeping your mind on your mat, so to speak, forces you to disengage from your stressors and to-dos for a little while. That can have a calming, quieting effect on your mind, even as your body is working hard.

Set a Time
AND STICK TO IT

Consistency really is the winning ticket when it comes to making progress in the fitness domain. Put your Pilates workouts on your calendar and treat them like important meetings or appointments. (Because as far as your health and quality

of life goes, they are!) I like to check my workouts off on the calendar as I complete them—there's something so satisfying about ticking that box. All of these workouts should take around 30 minutes, so you can slot yours in anytime—before heading out for the day, after you get home from work, or whenever feels most natural to you.

Rally
YOUR SUPPORT TEAM

We all have those days when it's tough to make yourself work out, even though you know you should. When you hit that wall, reach out to someone who'll give you a boost of encouragement. It just might be the push you need to stay on track.

A friend of mine was trying to keep up with his Pilates workouts while his wife underwent cancer treatments, and he was worried he might not stay motivated. So he asked me to hold him accountable. Each day he'd send me a quick text letting me know he'd completed his workout. And on the days I didn't get a message, I texted him to make sure he'd exercised that day. It worked, and he was able to reap the physical and mental benefits of a regular Pilates practice. He has told me over and over how this practice gave him energy and emotional balance. The stress of being a caregiver is incredible. Watching how the method helped him through this time confirmed my belief in the

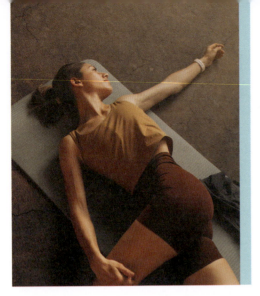

benefits of the work, both mental and physical. He has continued with his practice and now even teaches his wife! His experience made me more enthusiastic about my own practice too. Try letting a friend or family member know about your fitness goals so you always have access to a morale boost when you need it.

Make Time
TO RELAX

I like to say that no matter how much stress you're feeling in life, you should be getting the same amount of relaxation for optimal health. A new workout taxes your body and mind, and adequate rest is a must to allow yourself time to recuperate. Make sure you're getting the sleep that you need each night so you have the energy to give tomorrow's workout your all. If you're new to exercise or are adding this to an exercise program you're already doing, consider carving out time for a little more sleep than usual.

Be
PATIENT

Last but not least, acknowledge that progress can sometimes be slow going. We've all heard the adage "Rome wasn't built in a day." It can take some time to truly get the hang of Pilates and have the movements feel like second nature. Stick with it. Even if some of the exercises feel a little complicated or clumsy at first, in time you'll come to your practice feeling comfortable and confident.

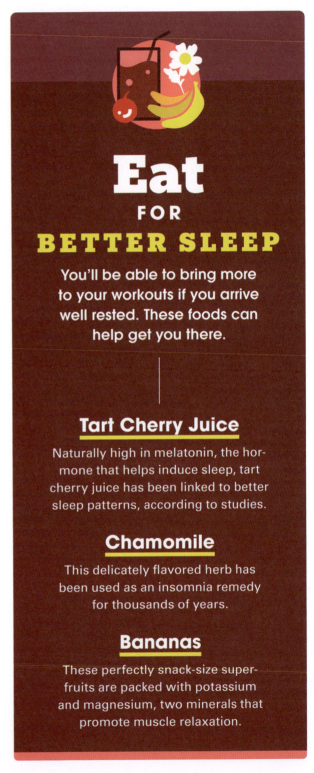

Eat
FOR
BETTER SLEEP

You'll be able to bring more to your workouts if you arrive well rested. These foods can help get you there.

Tart Cherry Juice

Naturally high in melatonin, the hormone that helps induce sleep, tart cherry juice has been linked to better sleep patterns, according to studies.

Chamomile

This delicately flavored herb has been used as an insomnia remedy for thousands of years.

Bananas

These perfectly snack-size superfruits are packed with potassium and magnesium, two minerals that promote muscle relaxation.

FIND YOUR
"Why"

Identifying the real reason you want to start this fitness journey can help you stay motivated even when sticking to the plan feels impossible. Use this space to reflect on why you want to make this change and revisit it when you're in need of a little motivation to keep going.

I want to start this plan because

By the end of this plan, I want to feel

03

How The Plan Works

IN TODAY'S BUSY WORLD, we're all shorter on time and attention than ever before. That can make it challenging to implement a new fitness routine filled with dozens of different exercises and daily workouts. That's why I've made this plan as simple and efficient as possible. I've cut down on any unnecessary work and left just the good stuff so it's easy to integrate this program into your life for the next 28 days and beyond. Every week you'll:

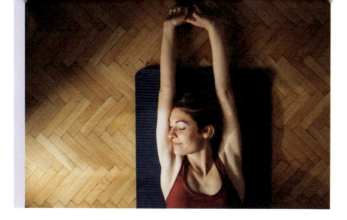

WORK OUT
FOUR DAYS

You don't need to hit the gym daily to boost your fitness. On this plan you'll work out just four days each week, resting a day between each workout to give your muscles time to recover (and give you time to attend to everything else in your life!). Every workout includes upper body, lower body, and ab exercises that'll help you get toned head to toe. Better yet, most exercises work multiple muscle groups at once, so you really are getting a total-body workout every time you hit the mat.

FOCUS ON
ONE SERIES
OF EXERCISES

Instead of varying your workouts throughout the week, you'll repeat the same series of 11 exercises for all four workouts. You know the saying—practice makes perfect! Repetition also limits the number of exercises you'll need to learn in a week, ensuring you can give all your attention to mastering the moves and getting results faster.

MAKE SMALL CHANGES
FOR BIG RESULTS

My final time-saver? Every exercise in this plan is a variation of 11 base exercises that you'll do in Week 1. Instead of learning dozens of completely different exercises throughout the next 28 days, you'll simply learn the 11 base moves, then make a small change to how you do each move every week. You might position your legs differently or add an extra step, but it will always build upon the exercise you already learned in Week 1. For example, in Week 1 you'll do the hundred with your legs bent 90 degrees. In Week 2, you'll do the hundred with your legs bent 45 degrees. In Weeks 3

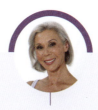

MY GOAL WITH THIS BOOK is to make regular exercise as easy as possible for you. Part of that is making sure you feel prepared for movement every time you get on your mat. As mentioned in Chapter 2, I'm providing a single warmup and cooldown to use before and after every workout (which you'll find starting on page 28). These moves will help you transition your body in and out of your workout, priming your muscles for movement and decreasing your chances of injuring yourself during your workout. I've also added breathing cues throughout most of the exercises to help you progress through the motions with ease. Aligning your inhales and exhales with particular movements in an exercise can provide a calming effect and even make strenuous movements feel a bit easier.

and 4, you'll do it with your legs straight. These simple variations help you gradually build your way to more challenging moves while continually sculpting lean muscle all over. You'll be impressed by how much your strength and flexibility will improve over just four weeks.

DO MORE
WHEN YOU FEEL READY

I've also included a series of 21 optional standing exercises. If you're up for a little more of a challenge, you can do these moves after finishing your workout for the day. Or, if you plan to repeat the 28-day program, you can add the standing exercises to your routine on your second go-around. These moves are designed to further strengthen and challenge your muscles, so add them in when you feel up to it!

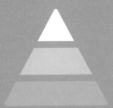

Elements of The Plan

In The 28-Day Workout Plan starting on page 26, you'll find everything you need to get toned head to toe in a month. Here's what you'll see.

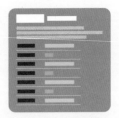

Week At-A-Glance

This zoomed-out view shows exactly what workouts you'll do each week and when you'll rest. Review it before starting your week so you can make time for exercise in your schedule.

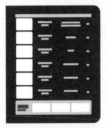

Workout Charts

Use the charts to find which exercises to do and for how many reps and sets. A rep is one run-through of all the steps in an exercise. A set is one round of all the reps listed in the "work" column. For full instructions and step-by-step photos, go to the page listed next to each exercise.

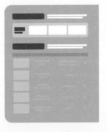

Daily Plan

Here's your roadmap for every day of the program. These pages list the week and day of the plan (days 1-28) you're on, so every day is a reminder that you're getting one step closer to your goal. Each indicates either a workout or a rest day.

Wellness Tracker

On each day's plan, you'll see a way to track some key elements of your health: how much water you drink, sleep you get, and how you feel. Here's why that's so important.

Hydration

Not getting enough water can sabotage your fitness efforts, with effects ranging from brain fog to fatigue. Track your daily water intake to make sure you're staying hydrated. Eight glasses a day is a great goal to aim for.

 Daily TRACKER

 WATER

 SLEEP

 MOOD

Sleep

Every task is more challenging when you're running on limited zzz's and that includes finding energy for a workout. Make note of when you go to bed and wake up each day—you might be logging less sleep than you need. Experts say adults need between seven to nine hours.

Mood

Over the course of 28 days most of us will experience a whole range of moods. Some may motivate us to give our workouts our best. Others, not so much. Jot down how you're feeling each day—you may notice patterns and eventually be able to course correct before a bad mood throws you off the path toward your goals.

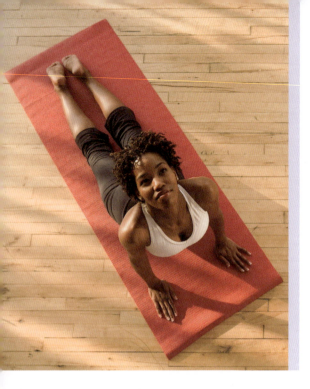

Adjusting the Plan to Your Fitness Level

We're all at different points in our fitness journey, which is why I've included multiple difficulty levels of each exercise. **Level 1 is the easiest; Level 2 is a little more challenging; Level 3 is the hardest.** You'll do Level 1 of each move in Week 1, Level 2 in Week 2, and Level 3 in Weeks 3 and 4.

Aim to follow the plan as I've laid it out, but listen to your body. If Level 1 of an exercise feels too easy by day 3, try Level 2. On the other hand, if Level 3 feels too difficult on day 15, stick with Level 2. You can be in different levels for different exercises to create a tailored plan that challenges you just the right amount.

Also: It's OK for an exercise to feel strenuous or hard, but it shouldn't hurt. Pushing yourself to the point of pain can set the stage for injury. So if an exercise seems to send up a flashing red light for your body, don't do it. And if you have any injuries or other health issues, consult with your doctor to make sure the moves in this plan are safe for you.

What Comes Next?

Completed your 28-day wall Pilates plan and wondering what you should do now? First, give yourself a pat on the back for a job well done. Then think about where you'd like to head next on your fitness journey.

You can repeat these exercises indefinitely if you'd like, redoing the program with your new insights and clarity. If things start to feel easy, add a few more repetitions or do all three levels of each exercise in every workout. (That'll really make you sweat.) You can also increase your tempo or pace to make the workout faster and add the standing exercises from pages 30 to 33.

If you've done the program a few times and are ready for a new challenge, consider attending an in-person Pilates class. You'll be prepared to tackle the more advanced exercises with your base movements down pat. Your instructor can help you further refine your form and alignment too.

Whatever path you choose, I hope this is the beginning of a new chapter of fitness and health in your life. **LET'S GET STARTED.**

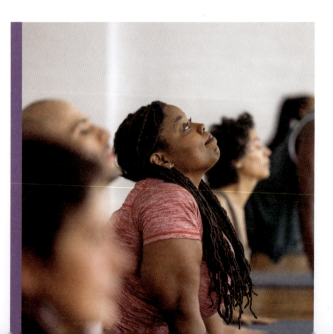

WHAT YOU'LL NEED

This wall Pilates workout incorporates all the same principles of the traditional Pilates method: **STRETCHING, STRENGTHENING, CENTERING, CONCENTRATING,** and **BREATHING WITH FLUID CONTROL AND PRECISION**. It supports healthy alignment and works your body from the inside out. The only difference? There's zero expensive equipment.

That said, you'll want to have a few basic items on hand. For the four-week plan, you'll need:

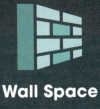

Wall Space

Wall Pilates

Comfortable Exercise Clothing

YOGA PANTS AND A STRETCHY TOP

A Thick Yoga Mat

WITH A TOWEL PLACED UNDERNEATH FOR EXTRA CUSHIONING

Optional Weights

FOR A CHALLENGE, USE TWO 1-LB WEIGHTS OR SOUP CANS

The 28-Day Workout Plan

Week 1 AT A GLANCE

Take things slow and steady this week to familiarize yourself with the base exercises of the program.

Monday	Level 1 Workout
Tuesday	Rest
Wednesday	Level 1 Workout
Thursday	Rest
Friday	Level 1 Workout
Saturday	Rest
Sunday	Level 1 Workout

Warmup Exercises

Complete this warmup before every workout in the 28-day plan to prepare your body for movement.

EXERCISE	WORK
Deep Breathing p. 74	**10 breaths**
Arm Arc Front p. 75	**3 - 5 reps**
Arm Arc Front 45 p. 76	**3 - 5 reps**
Arm Circle p. 77	**3 - 5 reps outward, 3 - 5 reps inward**
Hug With Elbow Lift p. 78	**3 - 5 reps per side**
Ankle Roll p. 79	**5 reps each direction per side**

EXERCISE	WORK

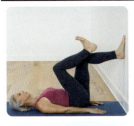

Flex and Point
p. 80

5 reps per side

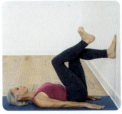

Toe Spread and Curl
p. 81

5 reps per side

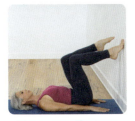

Toe Tap
p. 82

20 sec.

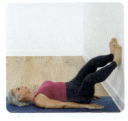

Windshield Wiper
p. 83

5 reps palms up,
5 reps palms down

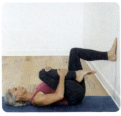

Single-Leg Stretch
p. 84

3 sec. per side

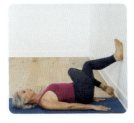

Cross-Leg Twist
p. 85

1 rep per side

Cooldown Exercises

Complete this cooldown after every workout in the 28-day plan to gradually transition your body out of exercise.

EXERCISE	WORK
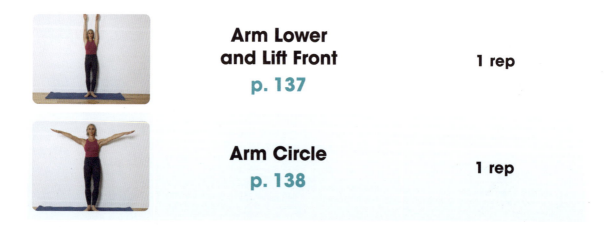 **Roll-Down With Arm Circle** p. 133	3 reps
Hug With Elbow Lift p. 134	1 rep per side
Lying With Legs Up The Wall p. 135	1 rep

Standing Exercises

Complete this optional series of standing exercises after any of your workouts if you'd like an added challenge.

EXERCISE	WORK
Arm Lower and Lift Front p. 137	1 rep
Arm Circle p. 138	1 rep

EXERCISE	WORK
Arm Curl p. 139	5 reps
Simple Roll-Down p. 140	3 reps
Roll-Down With Arm Circle p. 141	1 rep
Bend and Extend Knees p. 142	3 reps
Hands Rotate Down and Up p. 143	3 reps
Bend and Extend Knees With Shave p. 144	3 reps

Standing Exercises

Complete this optional series of standing exercises after any of your workouts if you'd like an added challenge.

EXERCISE	WORK
Side Bend 1 p. 145	**3 reps per side**
Side Bend 2 p. 146	**3 reps per side**
Side Bend 3 p. 147	**3 reps per side**
Book Covers p. 148	**3 reps per side**
Prayer p. 149	**3 reps per side**
Cat and Cow With Bent Knees p. 150	**3 reps**

EXERCISE		WORK
	Cat and Cow With Straight Knees **p. 151**	**3 reps**
	Curious Cat and Cow With Bent Knees **p. 152**	**3 reps**
	Extend and Bend **p. 153**	**5 reps per side**
	Extend and Bend: Foot on Wall **p. 154**	**5 reps per side**
	Extend and Bend: Foot on Wall With Heel Lift **p. 155**	**5 reps per side**
	Extend and Bend Squat **p. 156**	**5 reps**
	Single-Leg Extend and Bend Squat **p. 157**	**4 reps per side**

Week 1 | Day 1

Complete all exercises in the below Level 1 Workout chart, doing all sets of an exercise before moving on to the next exercise in the chart.

EXERCISE	WORK	SETS
The Hundred: Level 1 p.89	**20 reps head up, 20 reps head down**	**1**
The Roll Up: Level 1 p.93	**10 reps**	**3**
The One-Leg Circle: Level 1 p.97	**1 rep per side**	**1**
The Single-Leg Stretch: Level 1 p.101	**4 reps per side**	**1**
The Double-Leg Stretch: Level 1 p.105	**1 rep**	**3**
The Crisscross: Level 1 p.109	**3 reps per side**	**1**

EXERCISE	WORK	SETS
The Spine Stretch Forward: Level 1 p.113	**5 reps**	**1**
The Teaser Preparation: Level 1 p.117	**5 reps**	**1**
The One-Leg Kickback: Level 1 p.121	**3 reps per side**	**1**
The Side-Kick Series: Level 1 p.125	**1 rep per side**	**1**
The Spine Twist: Level 1 p.129	**5 reps per side**	**1**

Daily TRACKER

WATER

SLEEP
Bedtime Last Night
____:____
Wake Time This Morning
____:____

MOOD
☺ ☺ ☹

Week 1 | Day 2

Take this day to rest and use the Daily Tracker to record your water, sleep, and mood.

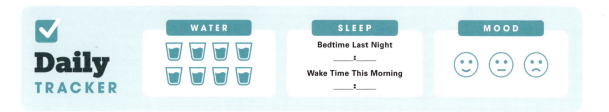

☑ **Daily** TRACKER

WATER	SLEEP	MOOD
🥛🥛🥛🥛 🥛🥛🥛🥛	Bedtime Last Night ____:____ Wake Time This Morning ____:____	🙂 😐 🙁

Week 1 | Day 3

Complete all exercises in the below Level 1 Workout chart, doing all sets of an exercise before moving on to the next exercise in the chart.

EXERCISE	WORK	SETS
The Hundred: Level 1 p.89	**20 reps head up, 20 reps head down**	1
The Roll Up: Level 1 p.93	**10 reps**	3
The One-Leg Circle: Level 1 p.97	**1 rep per side**	1
The Single-Leg Stretch: Level 1 p.101	**4 reps per side**	1
The Double-Leg Stretch: Level 1 p.105	**1 rep**	3

EXERCISE	WORK	SETS
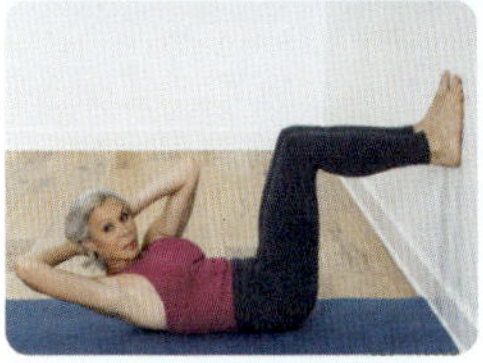 **The Crisscross: Level 1** p.109	**3 reps per side**	1
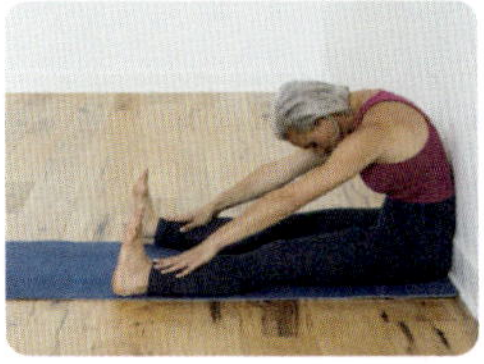 **The Spine Stretch Forward: Level 1** p.113	**5 reps**	1
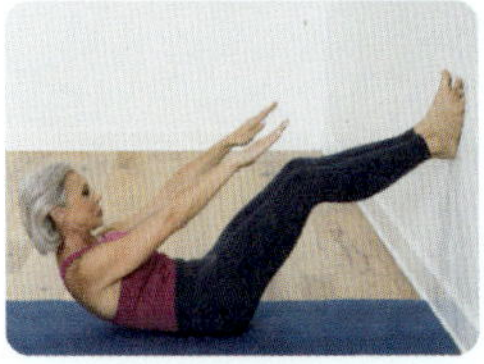 **The Teaser Preparation: Level 1** p.117	**5 reps**	1
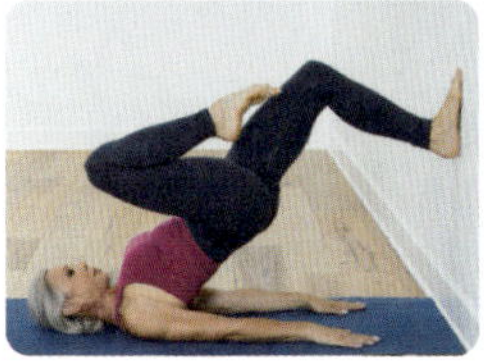 **The One-Leg Kickback: Level 1** p.121	**3 reps per side**	1
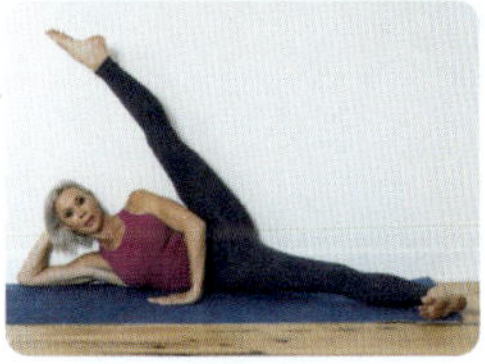 **The Side-Kick Series: Level 1** p.125	**1 rep per side**	1
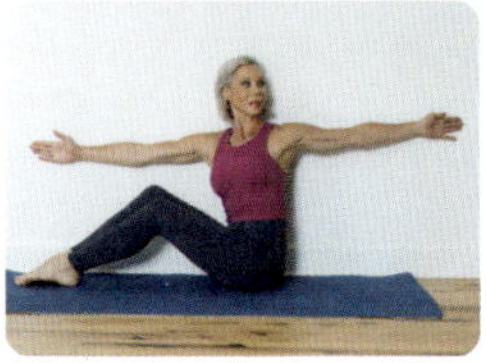 **The Spine Twist: Level 1** p.129	**5 reps per side**	1

☑️ **Daily** TRACKER

WATER

SLEEP
Bedtime Last Night
_____:_____
Wake Time This Morning
_____:_____

MOOD
🙂 😐 🙁

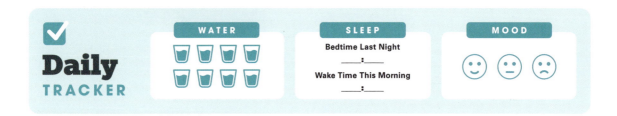

Week 1 | Day 4

Take this day to rest and use the Daily Tracker to record your water, sleep, and mood.

✓ **Daily** TRACKER

WATER

SLEEP
Bedtime Last Night
____:____
Wake Time This Morning
____:____

MOOD
☺ 😐 ☹

Week 1 | Day 5

Complete all exercises in the below Level 1 Workout chart, doing all sets of an exercise before moving on to the next exercise in the chart.

EXERCISE	WORK	SETS
The Hundred: Level 1 p.89	**20 reps head up, 20 reps head down**	1
The Roll Up: Level 1 p.93	**10 reps**	3
The One-Leg Circle: Level 1 p.97	**1 rep per side**	1
The Single-Leg Stretch: Level 1 p.101	**4 reps per side**	1
The Double-Leg Stretch: Level 1 p.105	**1 rep**	3

EXERCISE	WORK	SETS
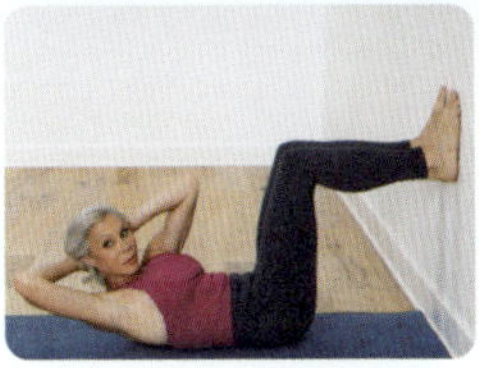 **The Crisscross: Level 1** p.109	3 reps per side	1
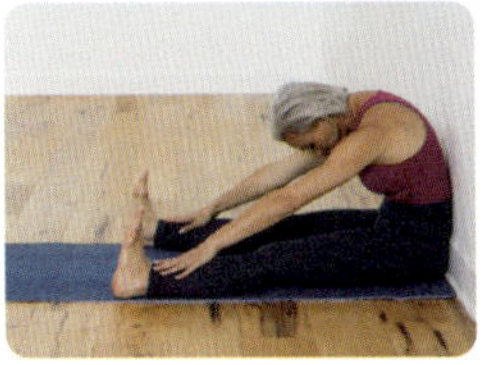 **The Spine Stretch Forward: Level 1** p.113	5 reps	1
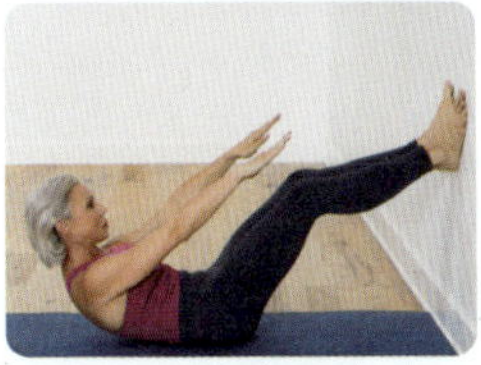 **The Teaser Preparation: Level 1** p.117	5 reps	1
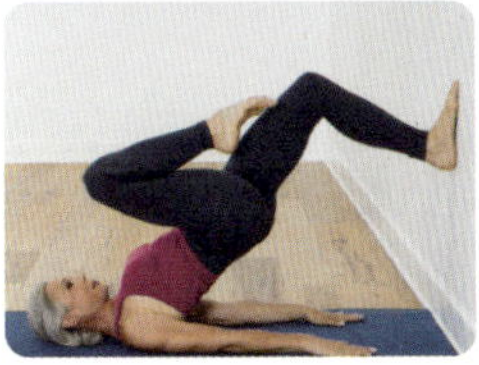 **The One-Leg Kickback: Level 1** p.121	3 reps per side	1
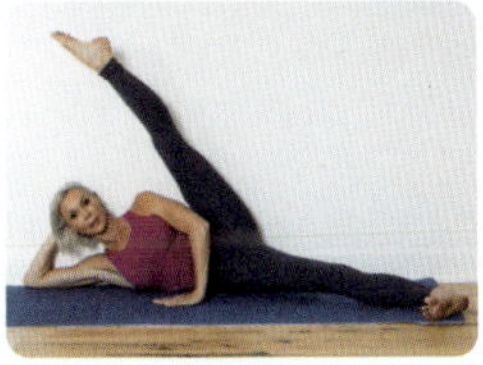 **The Side-Kick Series: Level 1** p.125	1 rep per side	1
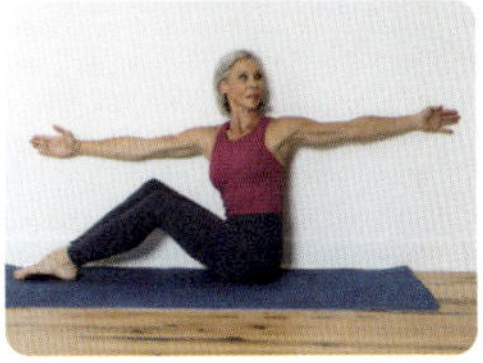 **The Spine Twist: Level 1** p.129	5 reps per side	1

☑ **Daily** TRACKER

WATER

SLEEP
Bedtime Last Night
_____:_____
Wake Time This Morning
_____:_____

MOOD
:) :| :(

Week 1 | Day 6

Take this day to rest and use the Daily Tracker to record your water, sleep, and mood.

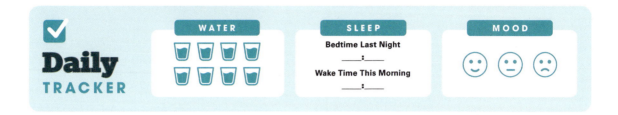

✓ **Daily** TRACKER

WATER

SLEEP
Bedtime Last Night
____:____
Wake Time This Morning
____:____

MOOD

Week 1 | Day 7

Complete all exercises in the below Level 1 Workout chart, doing all sets of an exercise before moving on to the next exercise in the chart.

EXERCISE	WORK	SETS
The Hundred: Level 1 p.89	**20 reps head up, 20 reps head down**	1
The Roll Up: Level 1 p.93	**10 reps**	3
The One-Leg Circle: Level 1 p.97	**1 rep per side**	1
The Single-Leg Stretch: Level 1 p.101	**4 reps per side**	1
The Double-Leg Stretch: Level 1 p.105	**1 rep**	3

EXERCISE		WORK	SETS
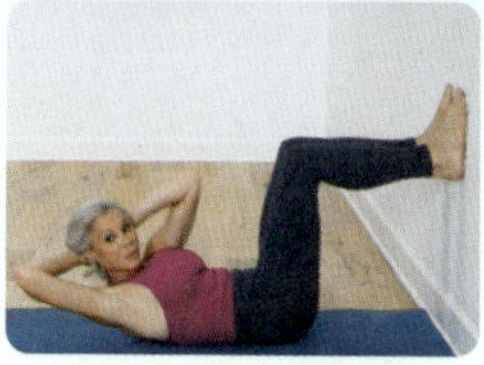	**The Crisscross: Level 1** p.109	3 reps per side	1
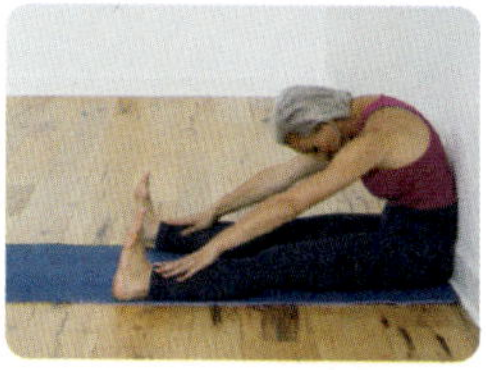	**The Spine Stretch Forward: Level 1** p.113	5 reps	1
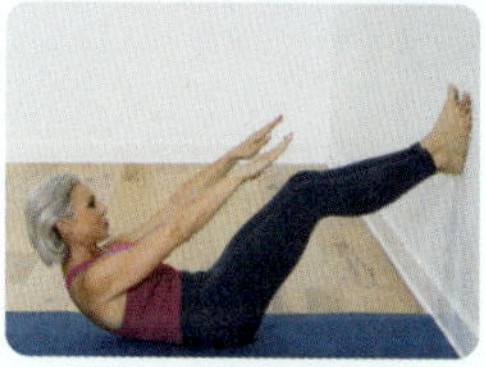	**The Teaser Preparation: Level 1** p.117	5 reps	1
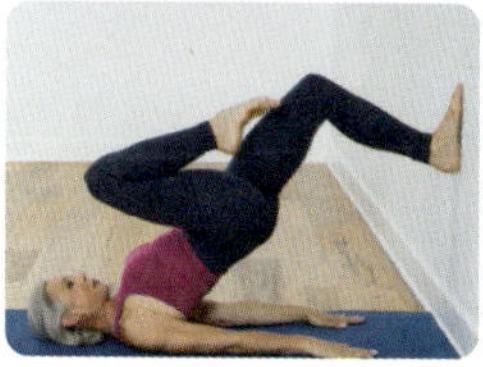	**The One-Leg Kickback: Level 1** p.121	3 reps per side	1
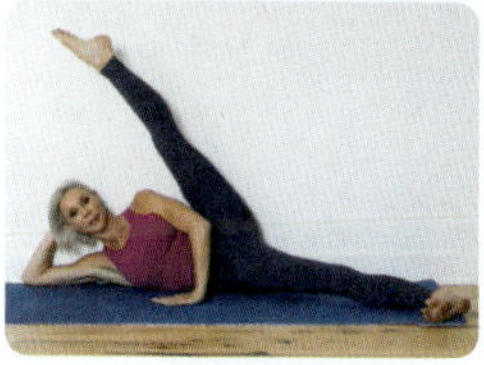	**The Side-Kick Series: Level 1** p.125	1 rep per side	1
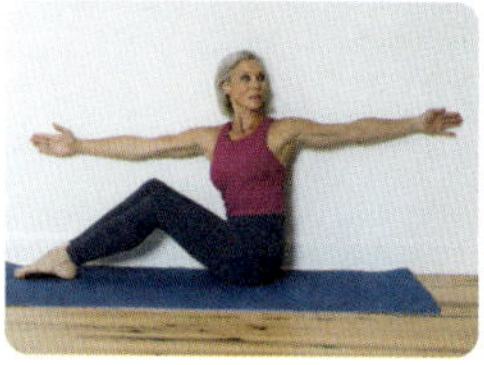	**The Spine Twist: Level 1** p.129	5 reps per side	1

✓ **Daily** TRACKER

WATER

SLEEP
Bedtime Last Night
_____:_____
Wake Time This Morning
_____:_____

MOOD
🙂 😐 🙁

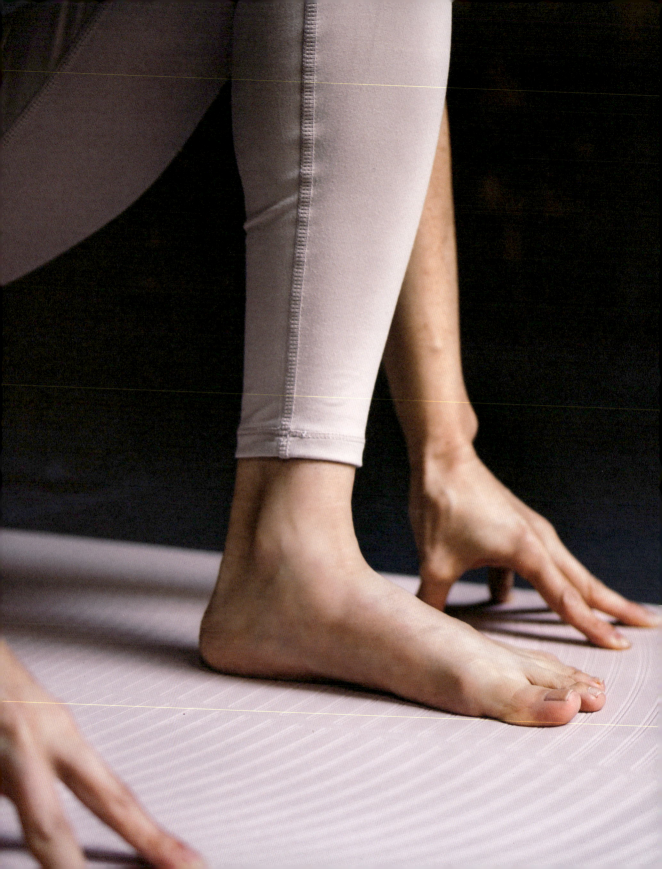

Week 2 AT A GLANCE

It's time to shake things up! This week you'll do slight variations of last week's exercises, giving you even greater toning benefits.

Monday	**Level 2 Workout**
Tuesday	**Rest**
Wednesday	**Level 2 Workout**
Thursday	**Rest**
Friday	**Level 2 Workout**
Saturday	**Rest**
Sunday	**Level 2 Workout**

Complete all exercises in the below Level 2 Workout chart, doing all sets of an exercise before moving on to the next exercise in the chart.

EXERCISE	WORK	SETS
The Hundred: Level 2 p.90	**30 reps head up, 30 reps head down**	1
The Roll Up: Level 2 p.94	**30 reps**	5
The One-Leg Circle: Level 2 p.98	**1 rep per side**	1
The Single-Leg Stretch: Level 2 p.102	**4 reps per side**	1
The Double-Leg Stretch: Level 2 p.106	**1 rep**	5
The Crisscross: Level 2 p.110	**3 reps per side**	1

EXERCISE	WORK	SETS
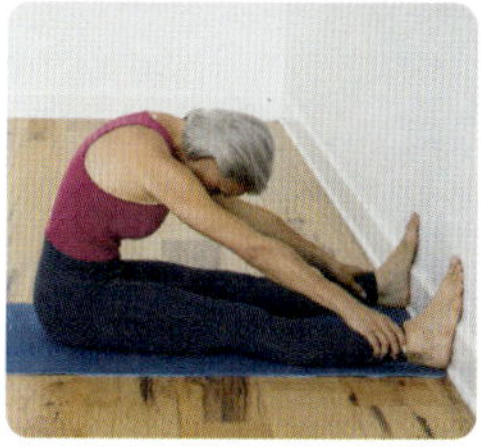 **The Spine Stretch Forward: Level 2** p.114	**5 reps**	**1**
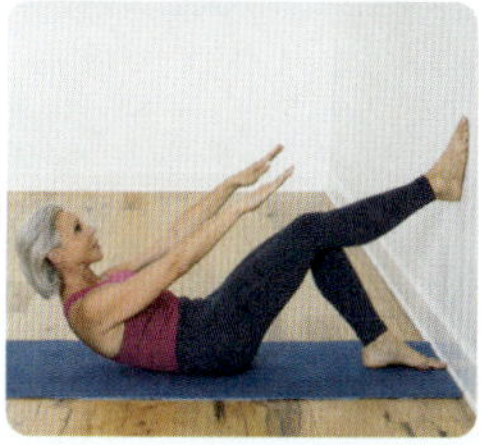 **The Teaser Preparation: Level 2** p.118	**5 reps**	**1**
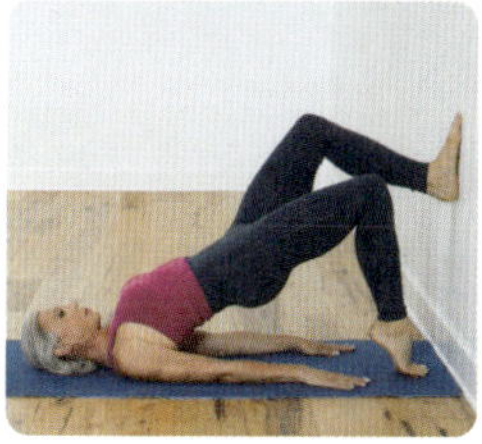 **The One-Leg Kickback: Level 2** p.122	**3 reps per side**	**1**
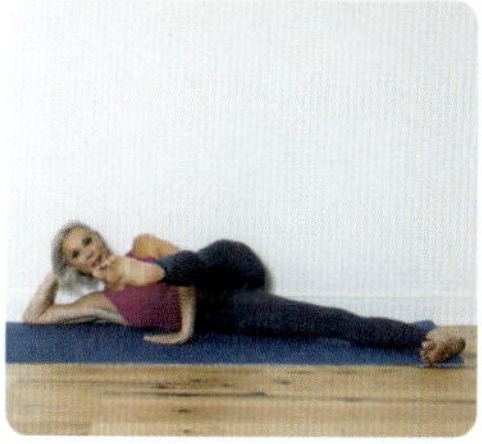 **The Side-Kick Series: Level 2** p.126	**1 rep per side**	**1**
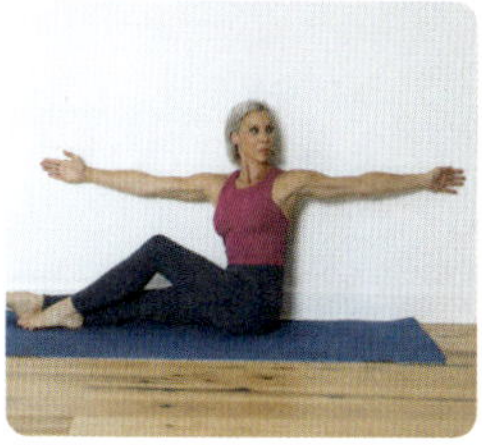 **The Spine Twist: Level 2** p.130	**5 reps per side**	**1**

Daily TRACKER

WATER

SLEEP
Bedtime Last Night
____:____
Wake Time This Morning
____:____

MOOD

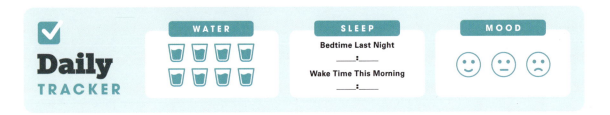

Week 2 | Day 9

Take this day to rest and use the Daily Tracker to record your water, sleep, and mood.

☑ Daily TRACKER

WATER

SLEEP
Bedtime Last Night
_____:_____
Wake Time This Morning
_____:_____

MOOD
☺ ☺ ☹

Week 2 | Day 10

Complete all exercises in the below Level 2 Workout chart, doing all sets of an exercise before moving on to the next exercise in the chart.

EXERCISE	WORK	SETS
The Hundred: Level 2 p.90	30 reps head up, 30 reps head down	1
The Roll Up: Level 2 p.94	30 reps	5
The One-Leg Circle: Level 2 p.98	1 rep per side	1
The Single-Leg Stretch: Level 2 p.102	4 reps per side	1
The Double-Leg Stretch: Level 2 p.106	1 rep	5

EXERCISE	WORK	SETS
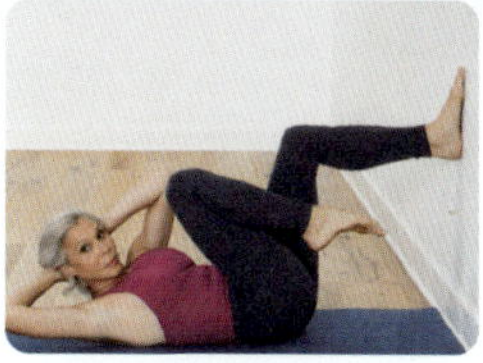 **The Crisscross: Level 2** p.110	3 reps per side	1
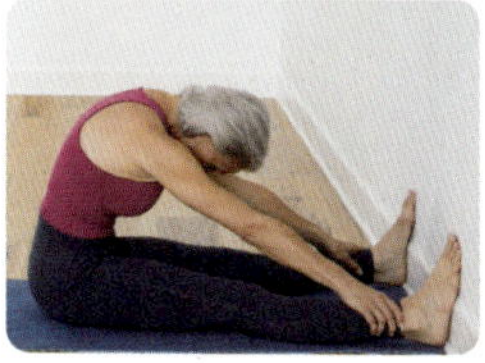 **The Spine Stretch Forward: Level 2** p.114	5 reps	1
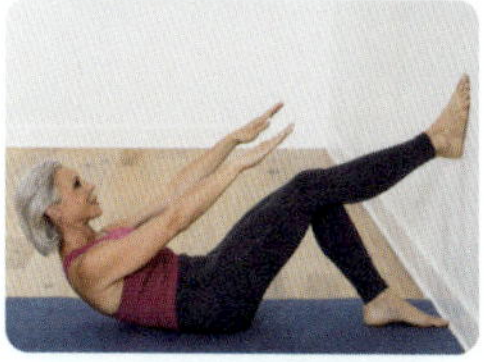 **The Teaser Preparation: Level 2** p.118	5 reps	1
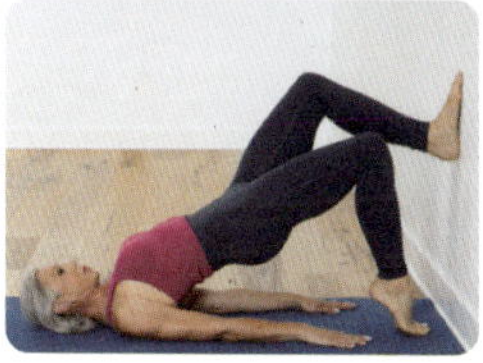 **The One-Leg Kickback: Level 2** p.122	3 reps per side	1
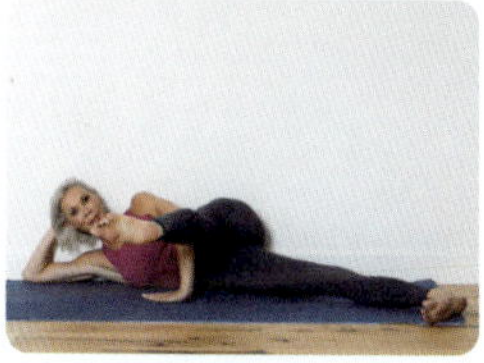 **The Side-Kick Series: Level 2** p.126	1 rep per side	1
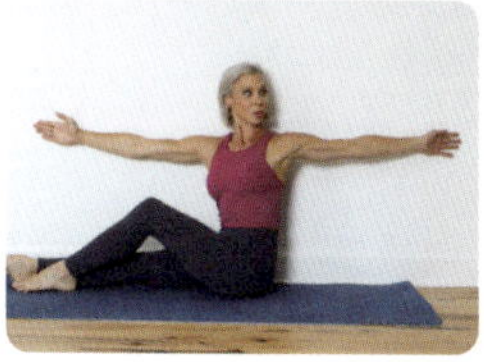 **The Spine Twist: Level 2** p.130	5 reps per side	1

✓

Daily TRACKER

WATER

SLEEP
Bedtime Last Night
_____:_____
Wake Time This Morning
_____:_____

MOOD
☺ 😐 ☹

Week 2 | Day 11

Take this day to rest and use the Daily Tracker to record your water, sleep, and mood.

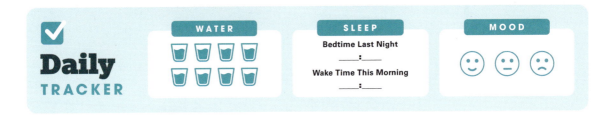

✔ Daily TRACKER

WATER

SLEEP
Bedtime Last Night
_____:_____
Wake Time This Morning
_____:_____

MOOD
☺ ☺ ☹

Week 2 | Day 12

Complete all exercises in the below Level 2 Workout chart, doing all sets of an exercise before moving on to the next exercise in the chart.

EXERCISE	WORK	SETS
The Hundred: Level 2 p.90	**30 reps head up, 30 reps head down**	1
The Roll Up: Level 2 p.94	**30 reps**	5
The One-Leg Circle: Level 2 p.98	**1 rep per side**	1
The Single-Leg Stretch: Level 2 p.102	**4 reps per side**	1
The Double-Leg Stretch: Level 2 p.106	**1 rep**	5

EXERCISE	WORK	SETS
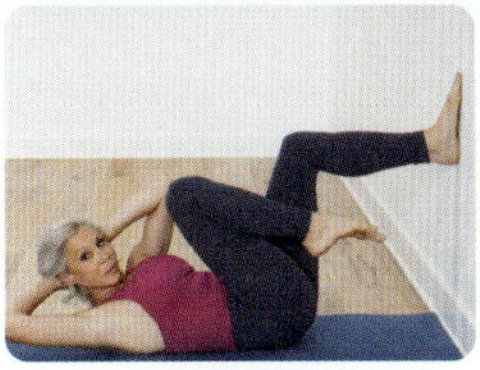 **The Crisscross: Level 2** p.110	3 reps per side	1
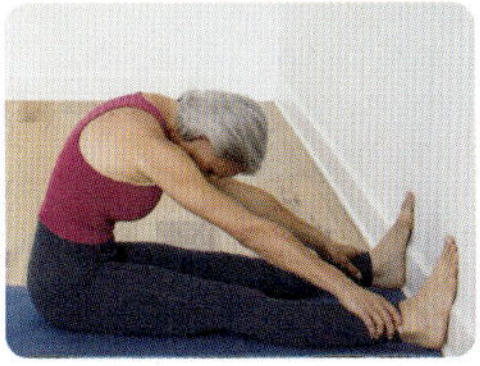 **The Spine Stretch Forward: Level 2** p.114	5 reps	1
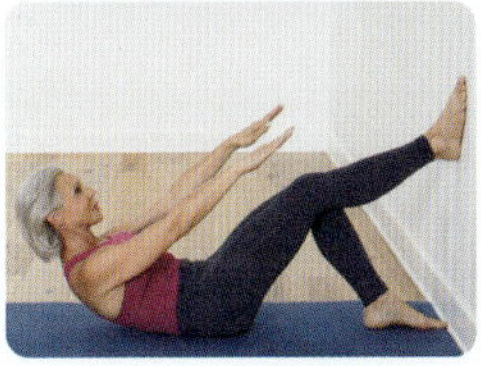 **The Teaser Preparation: Level 2** p.118	5 reps	1
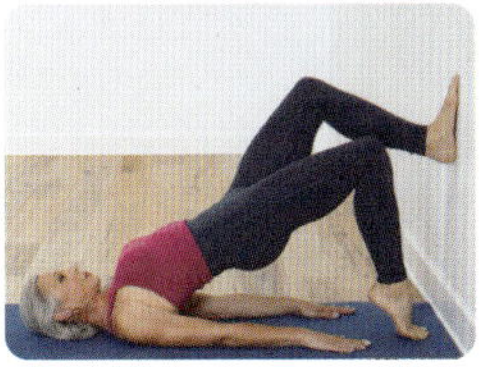 **The One-Leg Kickback: Level 2** p.122	3 reps per side	1
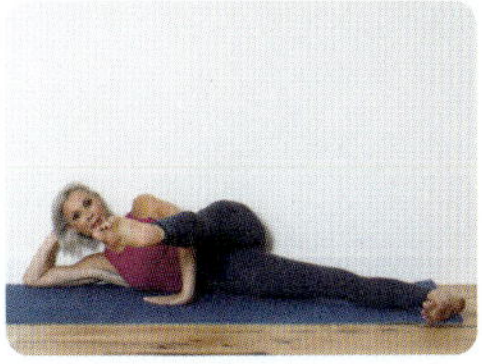 **The Side-Kick Series: Level 2** p.126	1 rep per side	1
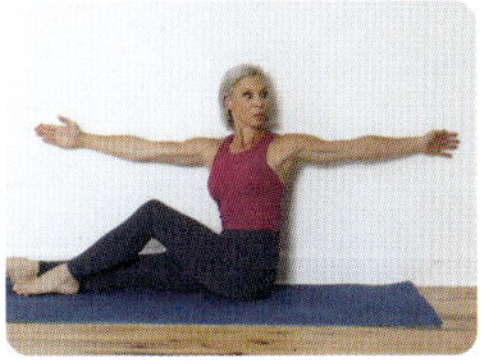 **The Spine Twist: Level 2** p.130	5 reps per side	1

☑️ **Daily TRACKER**

WATER

SLEEP
Bedtime Last Night
_____:_____
Wake Time This Morning
_____:_____

MOOD
🙂 😐 🙁

Week 2	Day 13

Take this day to rest and use the Daily Tracker to record your water, sleep, and mood.

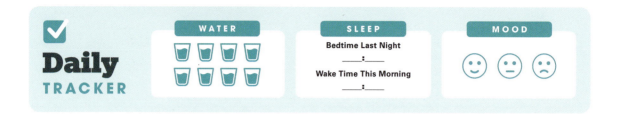

☑ Daily TRACKER

WATER

SLEEP
Bedtime Last Night
____:____
Wake Time This Morning
____:____

MOOD
☺ ☺ ☹

Week 2	Day 14

Complete all exercises in the below Level 2 Workout chart, doing all sets of an exercise before moving on to the next exercise in the chart.

EXERCISE	WORK	SETS
The Hundred: Level 2 p.90	30 reps head up, 30 reps head down	1
The Roll Up: Level 2 p.94	30 reps	5
The One-Leg Circle: Level 2 p.98	1 rep per side	1
The Single-Leg Stretch: Level 2 p.102	4 reps per side	1
The Double-Leg Stretch: Level 2 p.106	1 rep	5

EXERCISE	WORK	SETS
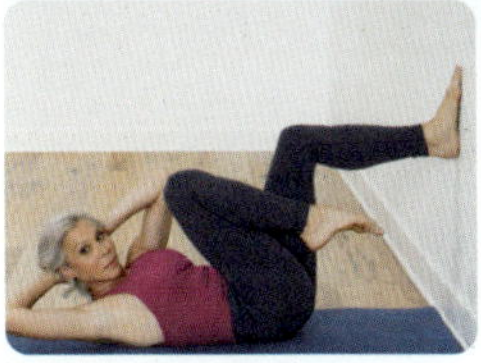 **The Crisscross: Level 2** p.110	**3 reps per side**	**1**
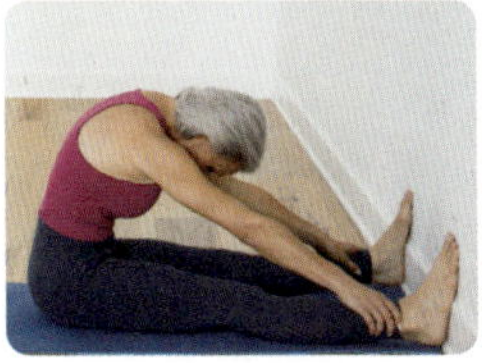 **The Spine Stretch Forward: Level 2** p.114	**5 reps**	**1**
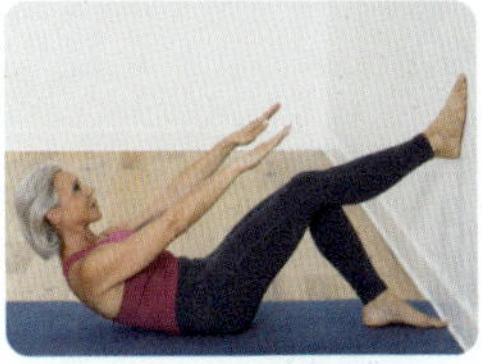 **The Teaser Preparation: Level 2** p.118	**5 reps**	**1**
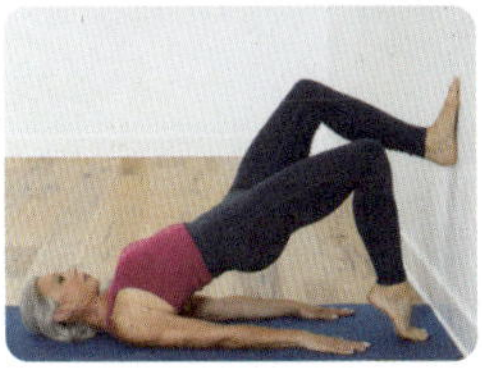 **The One-Leg Kickback: Level 2** p.122	**3 reps per side**	**1**
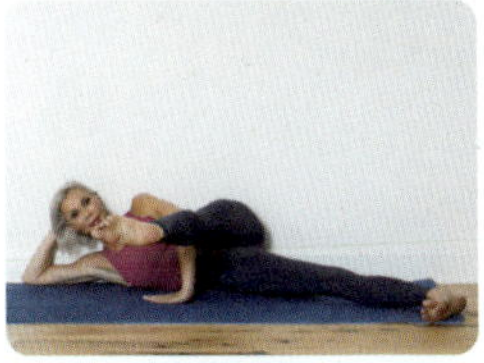 **The Side-Kick Series: Level 2** p.126	**1 rep per side**	**1**
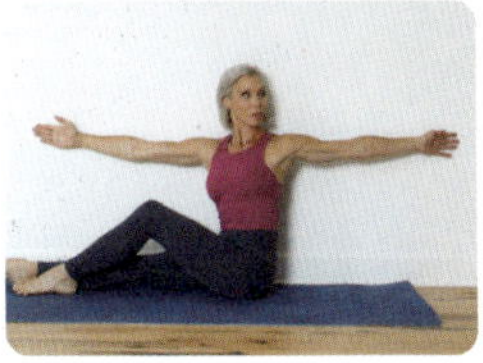 **The Spine Twist: Level 2** p.130	**5 reps per side**	**1**

Daily TRACKER

WATER

SLEEP
Bedtime Last Night
_____:_____
Wake Time This Morning
_____:_____

MOOD

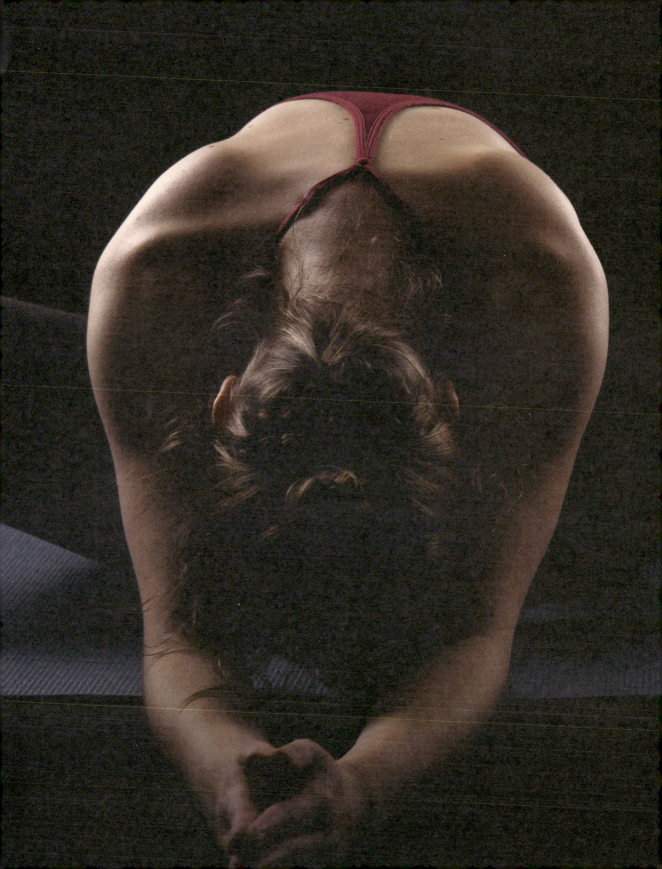

Week 3 AT A GLANCE

Ready for a little more? You'll do level 3 of all moves this week to build even more strength and boost your results. You've got this!

Monday	**Level 3 Workout**
Tuesday	**Rest**
Wednesday	**Level 3 Workout**
Thursday	**Rest**
Friday	**Level 3 Workout**
Saturday	**Rest**
Sunday	**Level 3 Workout**

Complete all exercises in the below Level 3 Workout chart, doing all sets of an exercise before moving on to the next exercise in the chart.

EXERCISE	WORK	SETS
The Hundred: Level 3 p.91	**10 reps**	**5**
The Roll Up: Level 3 p.95	**5 reps**	**1**
The One-Leg Circle: Level 3 p.99	**1 rep per side**	**1**
The Single-Leg Stretch: Level 3 p.103	**4 reps per side**	**1**
The Double-Leg Stretch: Level 3 p.107	**1 rep**	**5**
The Crisscross: Level 3 p.111	**3 reps per side**	**1**

	EXERCISE	WORK	SETS
	The Spine Stretch Forward: Level 3 p.115	**5 reps**	**1**
	The Teaser Preparation: Level 3 p.119	**5 reps**	**1**
	The One-Leg Kickback: Level 3 p.123	**3 reps per side**	**1**
	The Side-Kick Series: Level 3 p.127	**1 rep per side**	**1**
	The Spine Twist: Level 3 p.131	**5 reps per side**	**1**

☑ **Daily** TRACKER

WATER

SLEEP
Bedtime Last Night
_____:_____
Wake Time This Morning
_____:_____

MOOD
☺ 😐 ☹

Week 3 | Day 16

Take this day to rest and use the Daily Tracker to record your water, sleep, and mood.

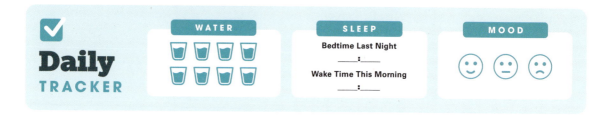

✔ **Daily** TRACKER

WATER

SLEEP
Bedtime Last Night
_____:_____
Wake Time This Morning
_____:_____

MOOD

Week 3 | Day 17

Complete all exercises in the below Level 3 Workout chart, doing all sets of an exercise before moving on to the next exercise in the chart.

EXERCISE	WORK	SETS
The Hundred: Level 3 p.91	**10 reps**	**5**
The Roll Up: Level 3 p.95	**5 reps**	**1**
The One-Leg Circle: Level 3 p.99	**1 rep per side**	**1**
The Single-Leg Stretch: Level 3 p.103	**4 reps per side**	**1**
The Double-Leg Stretch: Level 3 p.107	**1 rep**	**5**

EXERCISE	WORK	SETS
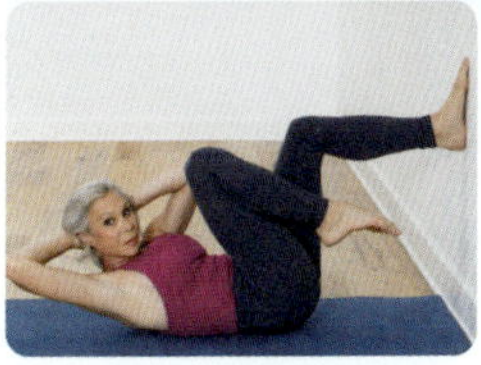 **The Crisscross: Level 3** p.111	3 reps per side	1
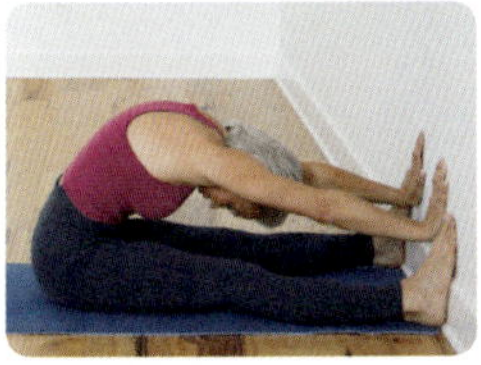 **The Spine Stretch Forward: Level 3** p.115	5 reps	1
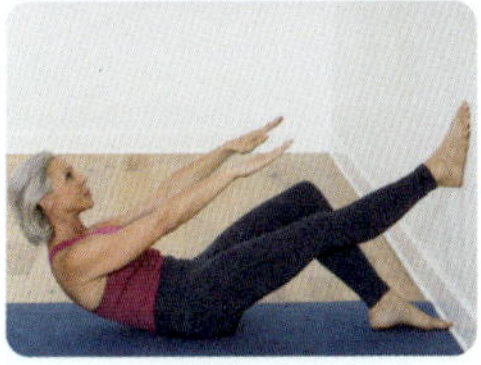 **The Teaser Preparation: Level 3** p.119	5 reps	1
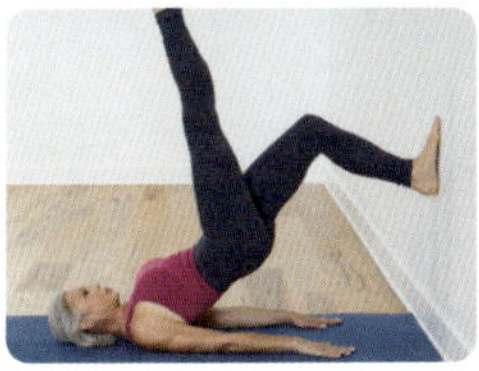 **The One-Leg Kickback: Level 3** p.123	3 reps per side	1
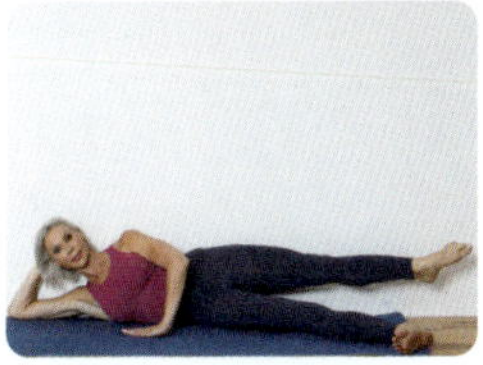 **The Side-Kick Series: Level 3** p.127	1 rep per side	1
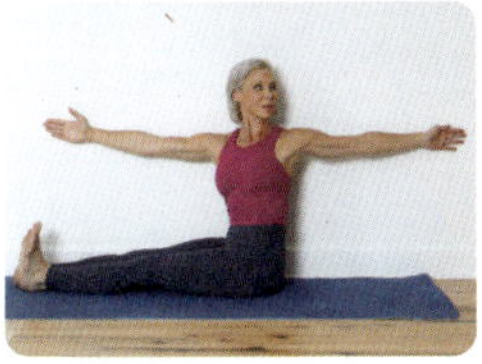 **The Spine Twist: Level 3** p.131	5 reps per side	1

✓ **Daily** TRACKER

WATER

SLEEP
Bedtime Last Night
_____:_____
Wake Time This Morning
_____:_____

MOOD
☺ ☺ ☹

Week 3 | Day 18

Take this day to rest and use the Daily Tracker to record your water, sleep, and mood.

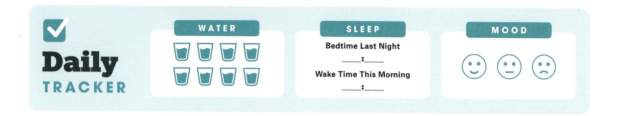

Daily TRACKER

WATER

SLEEP
Bedtime Last Night
____:____
Wake Time This Morning
____:____

MOOD

Week 3 | Day 19

Complete all exercises in the below Level 3 Workout chart, doing all sets of an exercise before moving on to the next exercise in the chart.

EXERCISE	WORK	SETS
The Hundred: Level 3 p.91	10 reps	5
The Roll Up: Level 3 p.95	5 reps	1
The One-Leg Circle: Level 3 p.99	1 rep per side	1
The Single-Leg Stretch: Level 3 p.103	4 reps per side	1
The Double-Leg Stretch: Level 3 p.107	1 rep	5

EXERCISE	WORK	SETS
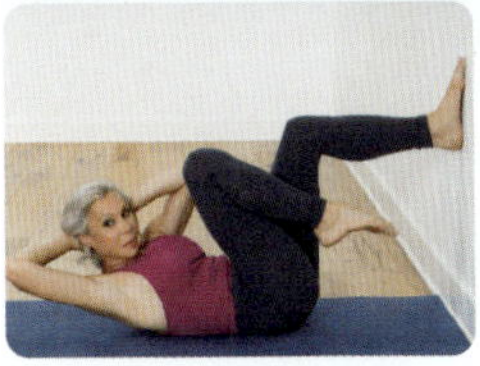 **The Crisscross: Level 3** p.111	**3 reps per side**	**1**
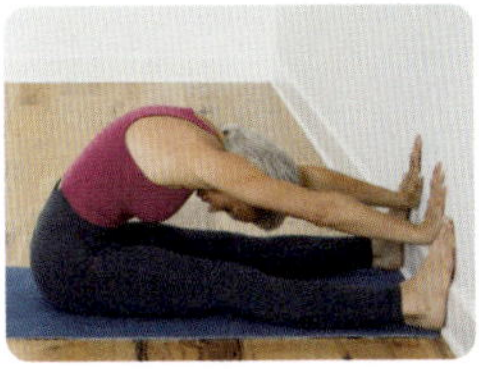 **The Spine Stretch Forward: Level 3** p.115	**5 reps**	**1**
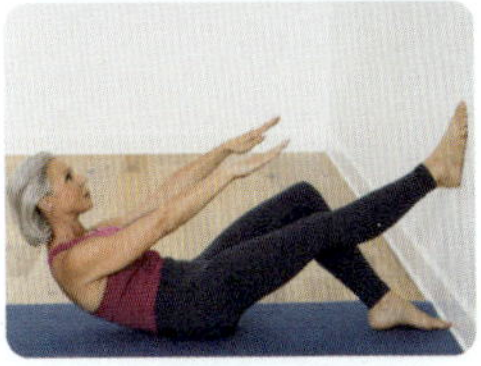 **The Teaser Preparation: Level 3** p.119	**5 reps**	**1**
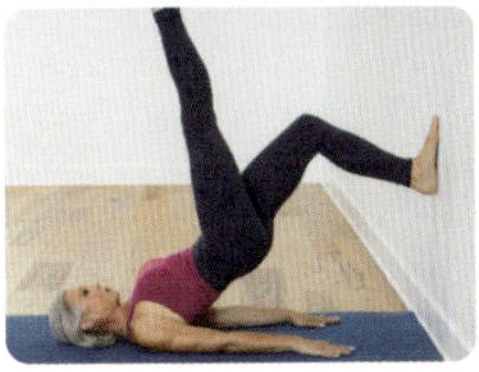 **The One-Leg Kickback: Level 3** p.123	**3 reps per side**	**1**
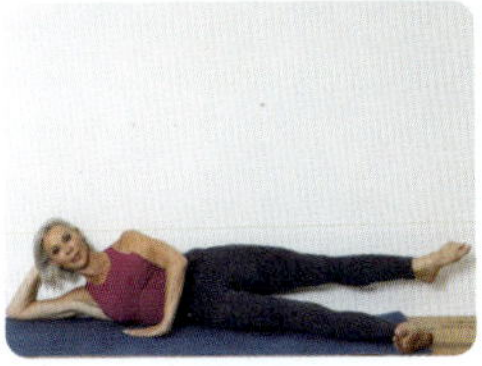 **The Side-Kick Series: Level 3** p.127	**1 rep per side**	**1**
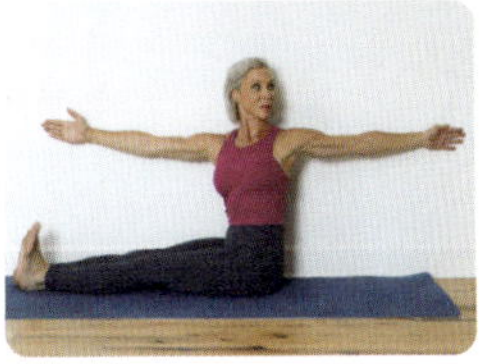 **The Spine Twist: Level 3** p.131	**5 reps per side**	**1**

✓ **Daily** TRACKER

WATER

SLEEP
Bedtime Last Night
_____:_____
Wake Time This Morning
_____:_____

MOOD
☺ ☺ ☹

Take this day to rest and use the Daily Tracker to record your water, sleep, and mood.

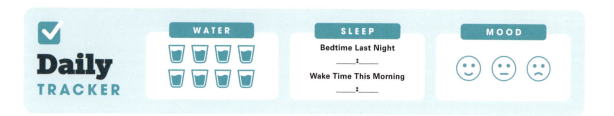

✓ **Daily** TRACKER

WATER

SLEEP
Bedtime Last Night
_____:_____
Wake Time This Morning
_____:_____

MOOD

Week 3	Day 21

Complete all exercises in the below Level 3 Workout chart, doing all sets of an exercise before moving on to the next exercise in the chart.

EXERCISE	WORK	SETS
The Hundred: Level 3 p.91	**10 reps**	**5**
The Roll Up: Level 3 p.95	**5 reps**	**1**
The One-Leg Circle: Level 3 p.99	**1 rep per side**	**1**
The Single-Leg Stretch: Level 3 p.103	**4 reps per side**	**1**
The Double-Leg Stretch: Level 3 p.107	**1 rep**	**5**

EXERCISE		WORK	SETS
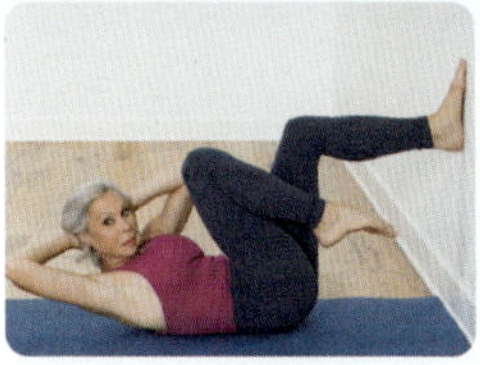	**The Crisscross: Level 3** p.111	3 reps per side	1
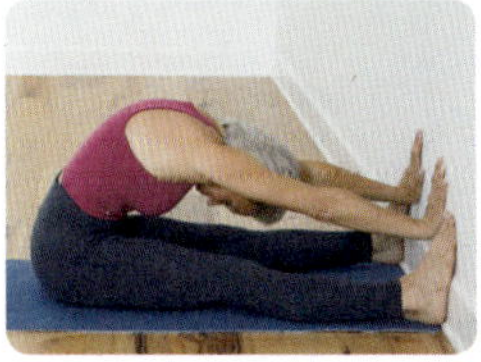	**The Spine Stretch Forward: Level 3** p.115	5 reps	1
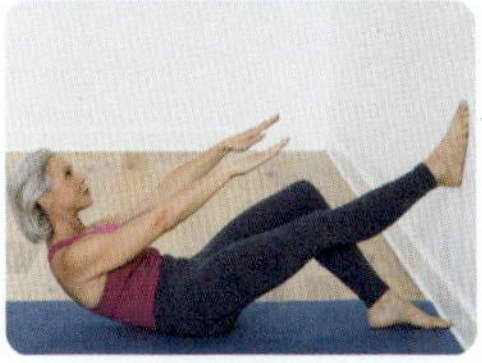	**The Teaser Preparation: Level 3** p.119	5 reps	1
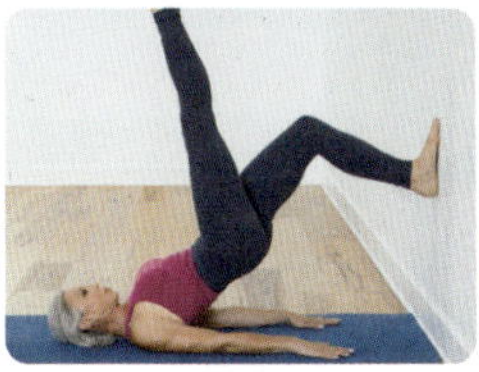	**The One-Leg Kickback: Level 3** p.123	3 reps per side	1
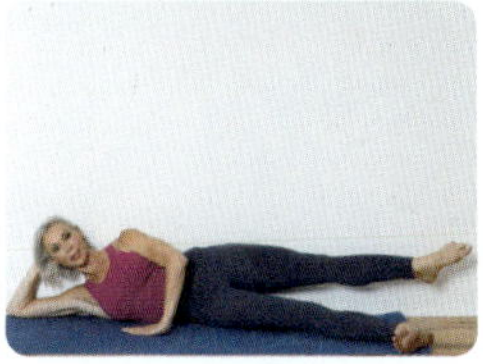	**The Side-Kick Series: Level 3** p.127	1 rep per side	1
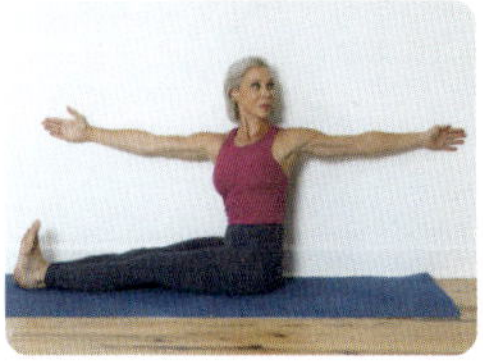	**The Spine Twist: Level 3** p.131	5 reps per side	1

✔️ **Daily** TRACKER

WATER

SLEEP
Bedtime Last Night
_____:_____
Wake Time This Morning
_____:_____

MOOD
🙂 😐 🙁

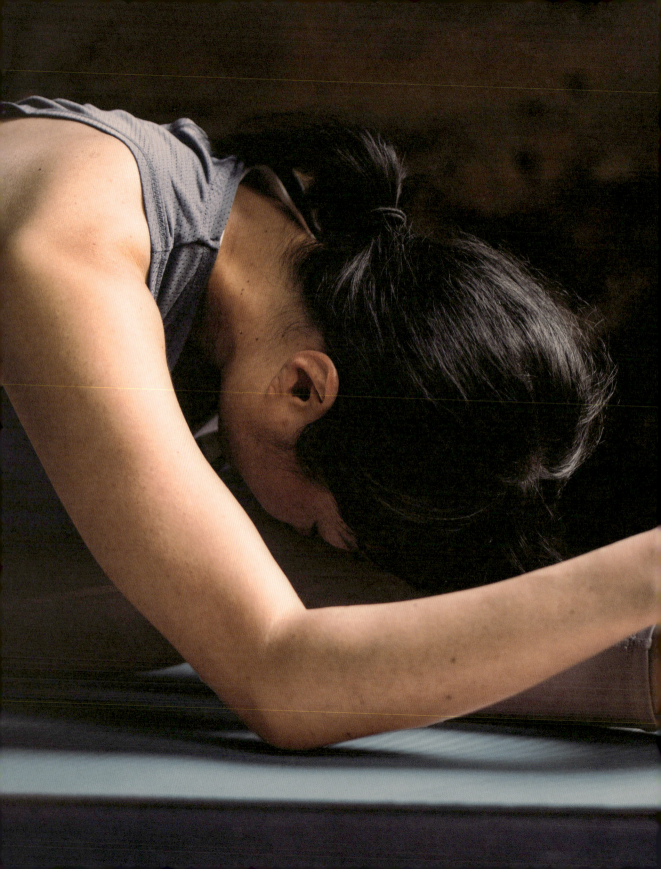

Week 4 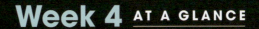 AT A GLANCE

You're almost there! For your final week of the plan, you'll repeat last week's workouts to perfect your form and finish strong.

Monday	**Level 3 Workout**
Tuesday	**Rest**
Wednesday	**Level 3 Workout**
Thursday	**Rest**
Friday	**Level 3 Workout**
Saturday	**Rest**
Sunday	**Level 3 Workout**

Complete all exercises in the below Level 3 Workout chart, doing all sets of an exercise before moving on to the next exercise in the chart.

EXERCISE	WORK	SETS
The Hundred: Level 3 p.91	**10 reps**	**5**
The Roll Up: Level 3 p.95	**5 reps**	**1**
The One-Leg Circle: Level 3 p.99	**1 rep per side**	**1**
The Single-Leg Stretch: Level 3 p.103	**4 reps per side**	**1**
The Double-Leg Stretch: Level 3 p.107	**1 rep**	**5**
The Crisscross: Level 3 p.111	**3 reps per side**	**1**

EXERCISE	WORK	SETS
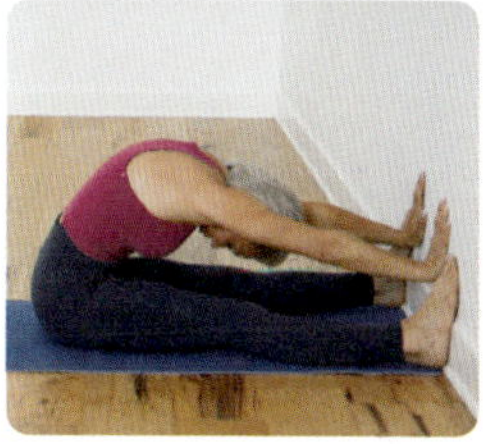 **The Spine Stretch Forward: Level 3** p.115	**5 reps**	**1**
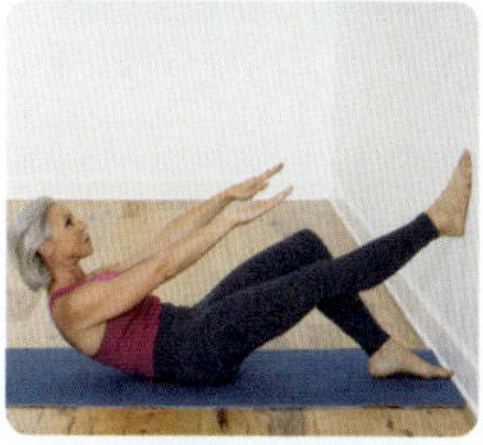 **The Teaser Preparation: Level 3** p.119	**5 reps**	**1**
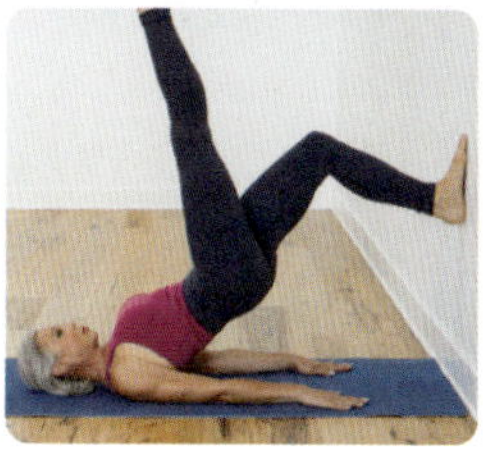 **The One-Leg Kickback: Level 3** p.123	**3 reps per side**	**1**
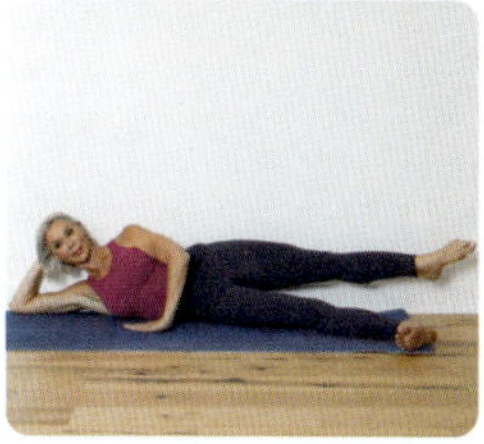 **The Side-Kick Series: Level 3** p.127	**1 rep per side**	**1**
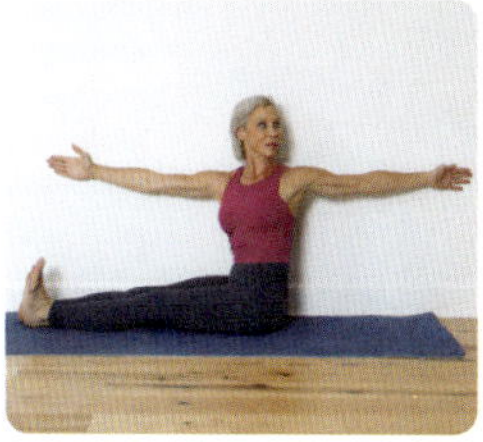 **The Spine Twist: Level 3** p.131	**5 reps per side**	**1**

✔️

Daily
TRACKER

WATER

SLEEP

Bedtime Last Night
____:____

Wake Time This Morning
____:____

MOOD

🙂 😐 🙁

Week 4 | Day 23

Take this day to rest and use the Daily Tracker to record your water, sleep, and mood.

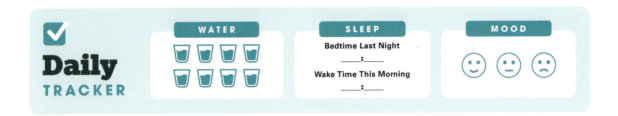

☑ **Daily** TRACKER

WATER

SLEEP
Bedtime Last Night
_____:_____
Wake Time This Morning
_____:_____

MOOD

Week 4 | Day 24

Complete all exercises in the below Level 3 Workout chart, doing all sets of an exercise before moving on to the next exercise in the chart.

EXERCISE	WORK	SETS
The Hundred: Level 3 p.91	**10 reps**	**5**
The Roll Up: Level 3 p.95	**5 reps**	**1**
The One-Leg Circle: Level 3 p.99	**1 rep per side**	**1**
The Single-Leg Stretch: Level 3 p.103	**4 reps per side**	**1**
The Double-Leg Stretch: Level 3 p.107	**1 rep**	**5**

EXERCISE	WORK	SETS
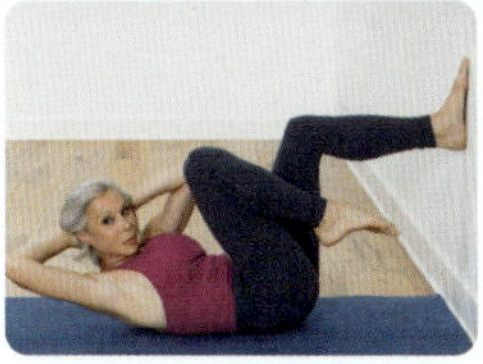 **The Crisscross: Level 3** p.111	3 reps per side	1
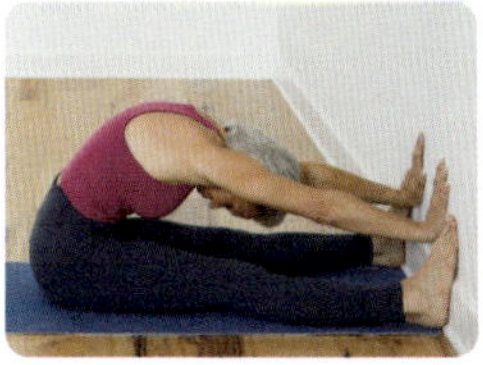 **The Spine Stretch Forward: Level 3** p.115	5 reps	1
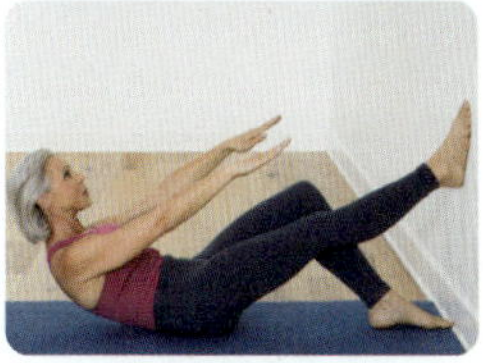 **The Teaser Preparation: Level 3** p.119	5 reps	1
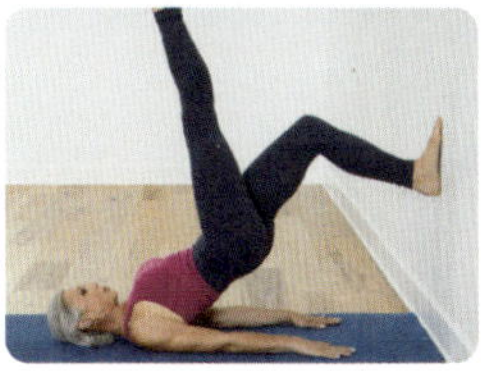 **The One-Leg Kickback: Level 3** p.123	3 reps per side	1
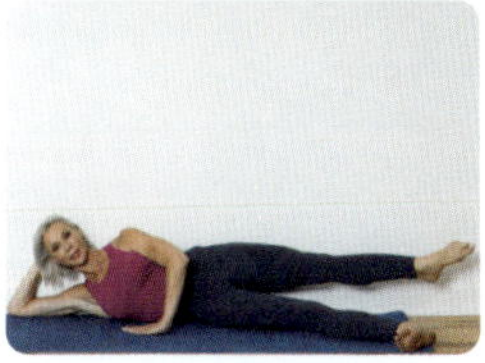 **The Side-Kick Series: Level 3** p.127	1 rep per side	1
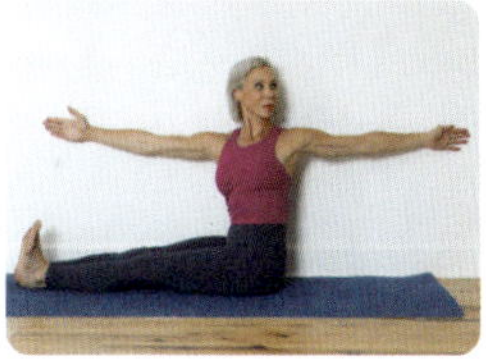 **The Spine Twist: Level 3** p.131	5 reps per side	1

✓ **Daily** TRACKER

WATER

SLEEP
Bedtime Last Night
____:____
Wake Time This Morning
____:____

MOOD
😊 😐 ☹️

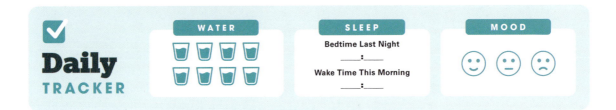

Week 4 | **Day 25**

Take this day to rest and use the Daily Tracker to record your water, sleep, and mood.

✓ **Daily** TRACKER

WATER

SLEEP
Bedtime Last Night
____:____
Wake Time This Morning
____:____

MOOD
😊 😐 🙁

Week 4 | **Day 26**

Complete all exercises in the below Level 3 Workout chart, doing all sets of an exercise before moving on to the next exercise in the chart.

EXERCISE	WORK	SETS
The Hundred: Level 3 p.91	**10 reps**	**5**
The Roll Up: Level 3 p.95	**5 reps**	**1**
The One-Leg Circle: Level 3 p.99	**1 rep per side**	**1**
The Single-Leg Stretch: Level 3 p.103	**4 reps per side**	**1**
The Double-Leg Stretch: Level 3 p.107	**1 rep**	**5**

EXERCISE	WORK	SETS
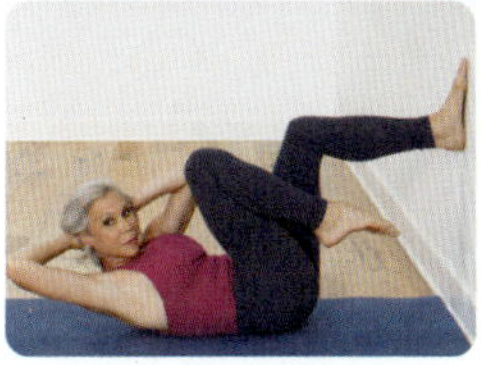 **The Crisscross: Level 3** p.111	3 reps per side	1
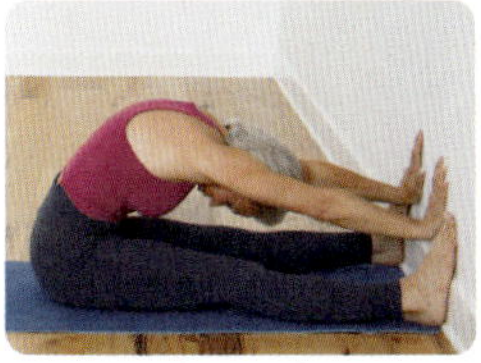 **The Spine Stretch Forward: Level 3** p.115	5 reps	1
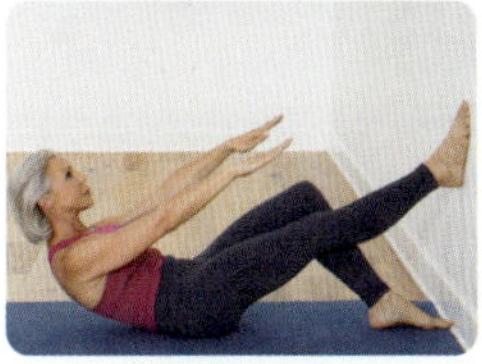 **The Teaser Preparation: Level 3** p.119	5 reps	1
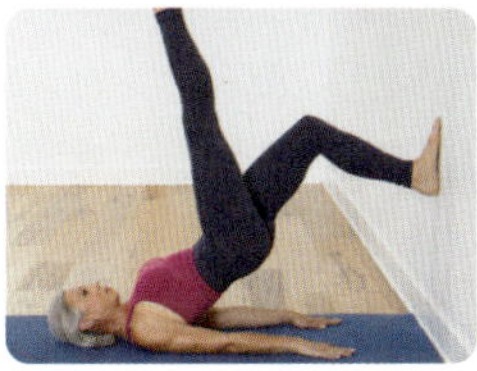 **The One-Leg Kickback: Level 3** p.123	3 reps per side	1
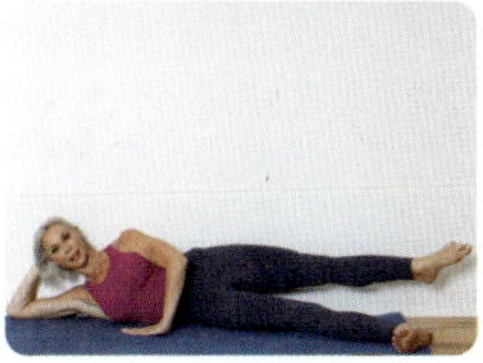 **The Side-Kick Series: Level 3** p.127	1 rep per side	1
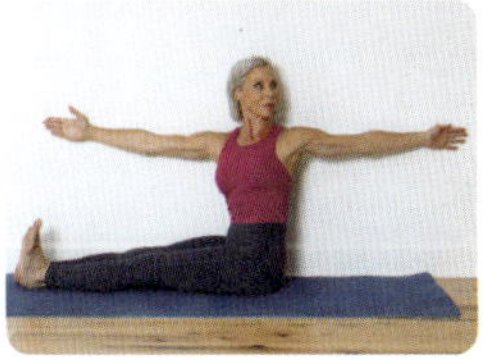 **The Spine Twist: Level 3** p.131	5 reps per side	1

✔️

Daily
TRACKER

WATER

SLEEP

Bedtime Last Night
____:____

Wake Time This Morning
____:____

MOOD

🙂 😐 🙁

Week 4 | Day 27

Take this day to rest and use the Daily Tracker to record your water, sleep, and mood.

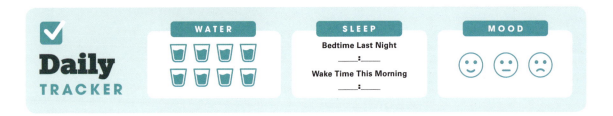

☑ **Daily** TRACKER

WATER

SLEEP
Bedtime Last Night
_____:_____
Wake Time This Morning
_____:_____

MOOD

Week 4 | Day 28

Complete all exercises in the below Level 3 Workout chart, doing all sets of an exercise before moving on to the next exercise in the chart.

EXERCISE	WORK	SETS
The Hundred: Level 3 p.91	**10 reps**	**5**
The Roll Up: Level 3 p.95	**5 reps**	**1**
The One-Leg Circle: Level 3 p.99	**1 rep per side**	**1**
The Single-Leg Stretch: Level 3 p.103	**4 reps per side**	**1**
The Double-Leg Stretch: Level 3 p.107	**1 rep**	**5**

EXERCISE	WORK	SETS
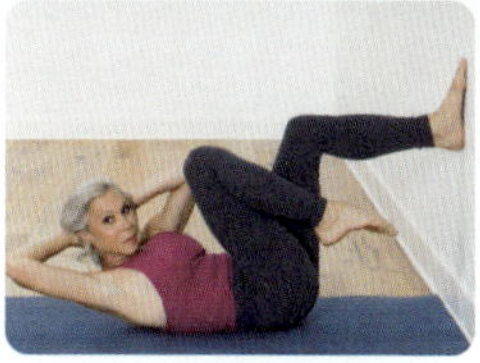 **The Crisscross: Level 3** p.111	3 reps per side	1
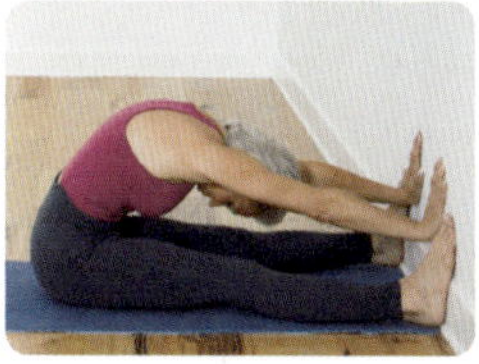 **The Spine Stretch Forward: Level 3** p.115	5 reps	1
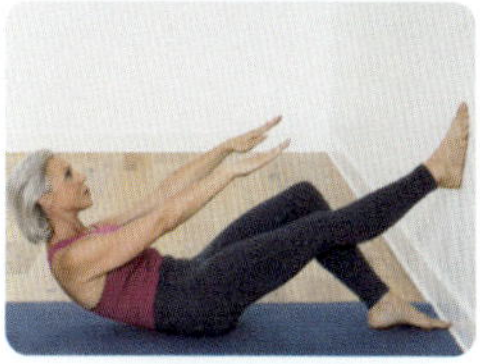 **The Teaser Preparation: Level 3** p.119	5 reps	1
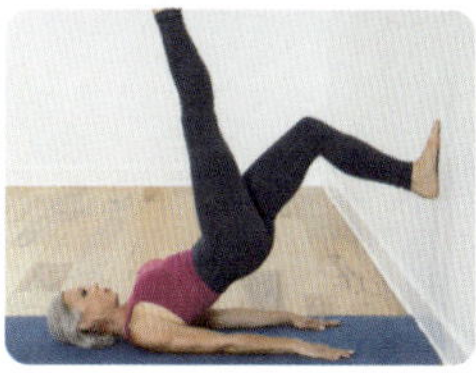 **The One-Leg Kickback: Level 3** p.123	3 reps per side	1
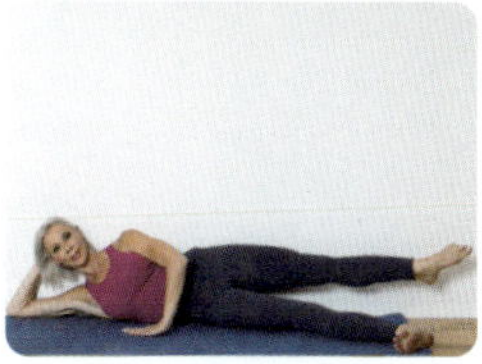 **The Side-Kick Series: Level 3** p.127	1 rep per side	1
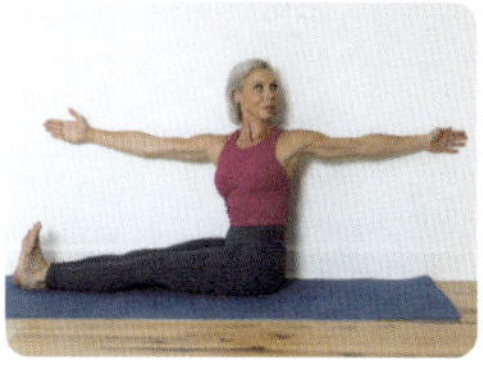 **The Spine Twist: Level 3** p.131	5 reps per side	1

✔️ **Daily** TRACKER

WATER

SLEEP
Bedtime Last Night
____:____
Wake Time This Morning
____:____

MOOD
🙂 😐 🙁

Exercise Glossary

PHRASES TO KNOW

Seeing results on this plan is all about prioritizing quality over quantity. Here's a breakdown of some phrases you'll see throughout the exercise glossary to help you master every move.

Arched Lower Back

When your lower back lifts off the floor as your pelvis tips its weight onto your tailbone.

Arched Neck

When your chin tilts up and its weight tips toward the crown of your head, shortening your neck.

Sit (or Sitting) Bones

Known collectively as your ischial tuberosity, these two bony points are found in the lower middle part of your buttocks and are what hurt when you sit on a hard chair.

Chin to Chest

In this position, your upper body rounds forward, leading with your head. Your gaze is toward your lower abdomen. Your throat remains long and your upper body rolls off the mat high enough to put the weight of your head into your abdominals and not in your neck.

Warmup

EXERCISES

Deep Breathing

Arm Arcs Front

Arm Arcs Front 45

Arm Circle

Hug with Elbow Lift

Ankle Roll

Flex and Point

Toe Spread and Curl

Toe Tap

Windshield Wiper

Single-Leg Stretch

Cross-Leg Twist

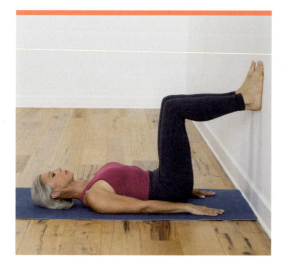

Deep Breathing

SETUP

Lie on a mat and place your feet flat on the wall hip-width apart, knees bent 90 degrees. Place your arms down by your sides. Keep your back long and flat to the mat.

STEPS

1 **INHALE DEEPLY** through your nose for 4 seconds. Hold your breath for 4 seconds.

2 **EXHALE FULLY** through your nose or mouth for 6 seconds. **HOLD AT THE BOTTOM OF THE LAST EXHALE** for 4 seconds. Continue for the prescribed amount of time.

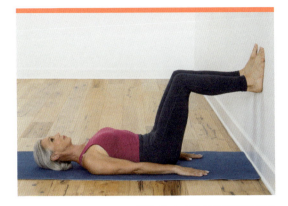

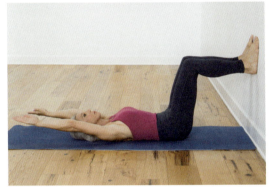

Arm Arc Front

SETUP

Lie on a mat and place your feet flat on the wall hip-width apart, knees bent 90 degrees. Place your arms down by your sides. Keep your back long and flat to the mat.

STEPS

1 **LIFT YOUR ARMS STEADILY** toward the ceiling and back over the top of your head as far as you can comfortably reach without arching your back. **WHILE LIFTING, INHALE DEEPLY** through your nose for 4 seconds. Hold your breath for 4 seconds.

2 Bring your arms back down toward your sides **WHILE EXHALING FULLY** through your nose or mouth for 6 seconds. That's 1 rep. Continue for the prescribed number of reps.

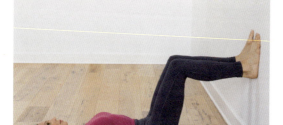

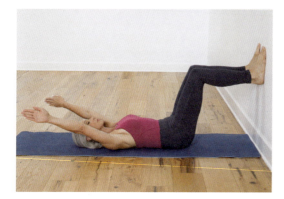

Arm Arc Front 45

Follow the same setup and steps as Arm Arc Front, but in Step 1 **LIFT YOUR ARMS IN A V SHAPE,** about 45 degrees out from your shoulders, instead of keeping your arms close to your body as you lift them toward the ceiling.

SETUP

Lie on a mat and place your feet flat on the wall hip-width apart, knees bent 90 degrees. Place your arms down by your sides. Keep your back long and flat to the mat.

STEPS

1 **LIFT YOUR ARMS STEADILY AT A 45-DEGREE ANGLE** toward the ceiling and back over the top of your head as far as you can comfortably reach without arching your back. While lifting, **INHALE DEEPLY** through your nose for 4 seconds. Hold your breath for 4 seconds.

2 **BRING YOUR ARMS BACK DOWN** toward your sides **WHILE EXHALING FULLY** through your nose or mouth for 6 seconds. That's 1 rep. Continue for the prescribed number of reps.

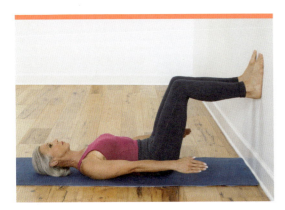

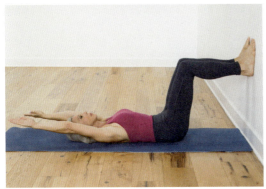

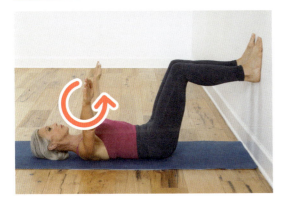

Arm Circle

Follow the same setup and steps as Arm Arc Front, but in Step 2 **OPEN YOUR ARMS TO THE SIDES TO MAKE A T SHAPE** instead of bringing them back to your sides. From here, make small outward circles with your arms as you lower them back to your sides.

SETUP

Lie on a mat and place your feet flat on the wall hip-width apart, knees bent 90 degrees. Place your arms down by your sides. Keep your back long and flat to the mat.

STEPS

1 **LIFT YOUR ARMS STEADILY** toward the ceiling and back over the top of your head as far as you can comfortably reach without arching your back. While lifting, **INHALE DEEPLY** through your nose for 4 seconds. Hold your breath for 4 seconds.

2 **OPEN YOUR ARMS OUT TO MAKE A T SHAPE WHILE EXHALING FULLY** through your nose or mouth for 6 seconds. Circle your arms back down to the starting position. That's 1 rep. Continue for the prescribed number of reps.

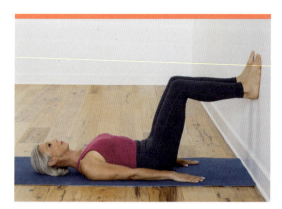

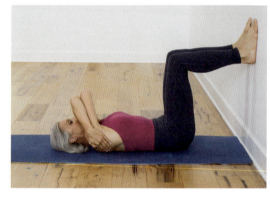

Hug With Elbow Lift

SETUP

Lie on a mat and place your feet flat on the wall hip-width apart, knees bent 90 degrees. Place your arms down by your sides. Keep your back long and flat to the mat.

STEPS

1 **CROSS YOUR ARMS OVER YOUR CHEST** as if you're giving yourself a hug. Reach each hand as far around your opposite shoulder blade as you comfortably can to get a nice stretch in your arms and shoulders. Try to keep your neck and tailbone flat on the ground.

2 **LIFT YOUR ELBOWS TOWARD YOUR NOSE,** inhaling for 4 seconds through your nose. **LOWER YOUR ELBOWS WHILE EXHALING** for 4 seconds through your nose. That's 1 rep. Continue for the prescribed number of reps; repeat with the opposite arm on top.

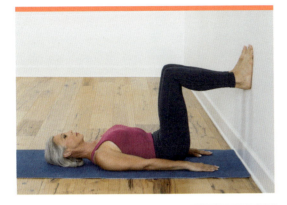

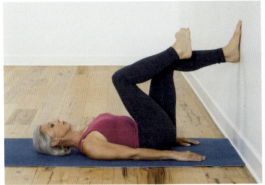

Ankle Roll

SETUP

Lie on a mat and place your feet flat on the wall hip-width apart, knees bent 90 degrees. Place your arms down by your sides. Keep your back long and flat to the mat.

STEPS

1 **BEND YOUR RIGHT KNEE** toward your chest, keeping your hip, knee, and ankle aligned. (Your knee doesn't have to touch.) **MAKE SLOW CLOCKWISE CIRCLES WITH YOUR RIGHT ANKLE** for the prescribed number of reps. Repeat, going counterclockwise for the prescribed number of reps. Try to keep your hips, knees, and ankles aligned as you make the circles. Place your right foot back on the wall.

2 Repeat with your left foot for the prescribed number of reps.

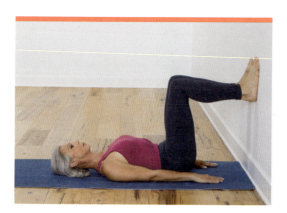

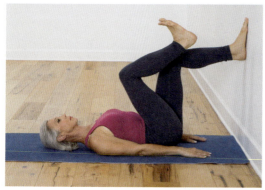

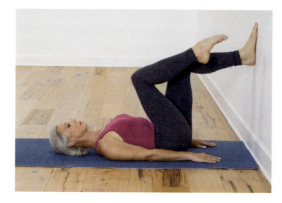

Flex and Point

Follow the same setup and steps as **ANKLE ROLL**, but in Step 1, **flex and point your right foot instead of circling it.**

SETUP

Lie on a mat and place your feet flat on the wall hip-width apart, knees bent 90 degrees. Place your arms down by your sides. Keep your back long and flat to the mat.

STEPS

1 **BEND YOUR RIGHT KNEE TOWARD YOUR CHEST,** keeping your hip, knee, and ankle aligned. (Your knee doesn't have to touch.) **FLEX AND POINT YOUR RIGHT FOOT,** spreading your toes while you flex. That's 1 rep. Continue for the prescribed number of reps, then place your right foot back on the wall and repeat on the left side.

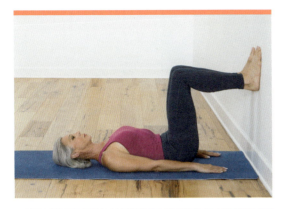

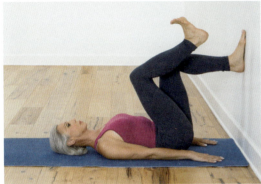

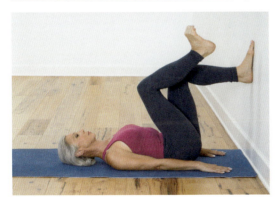

Toe Spread and Curl

Follow the same setup and steps as **ANKLE ROLL**, but in Step 1, **flex your right foot, spreading your toes open wide;** then curl your toes.

SETUP

Lie on a mat and place your feet flat on the wall hip-width apart, knees bent 90 degrees. Place your arms down by your sides. Keep your back long and flat to the mat.

STEPS

1 **BEND YOUR RIGHT KNEE TOWARD YOUR CHEST,** keeping your hip, knee, and ankle aligned. (Your knee doesn't have to touch.) **FLEX YOUR RIGHT FOOT, SPREADING YOUR TOES WIDE,** then curl your toes as if you're wrapping them around a pencil. That's 1 rep. Continue for the prescribed number of reps, then place your right foot back on the wall and repeat on the left side.

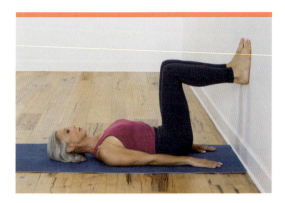

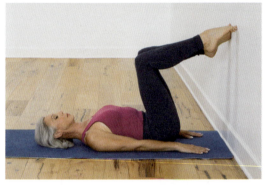

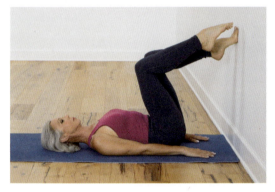

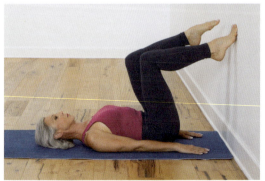

Toe Tap

SETUP

Lie on a mat and place your feet flat on the wall hip-width apart, knees bent 90 degrees. Place your arms down by your sides. Keep your back long and flat to the mat.

STEPS

1 **LIFT YOUR HEELS OFF THE WALL.** Alternating feet, **QUICKLY TAP THE BALLS OF YOUR FEET** to the wall for the prescribed amount of time. Try not to wiggle your hips or shoulders while you tap. **END WITH BOTH BALLS OF YOUR FEET ON THE WALL.**

2 Place your heels back on the wall and relax for 5 seconds.

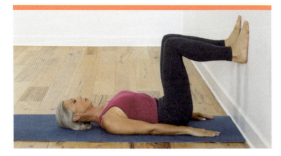
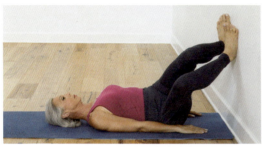
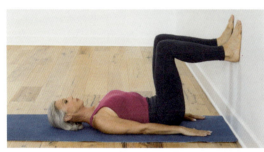
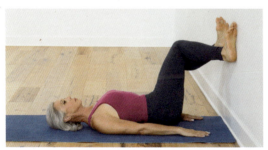
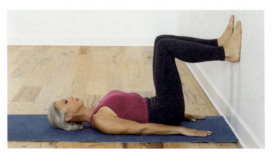

Windshield Wiper

SETUP

Lie on a mat and place your feet flat on the wall hip-width apart, knees bent 90 degrees. Place your arms down by your sides, palms down. Keep your back long and flat to the mat.

STEPS

1 **ROTATE YOUR HIPS AND KNEES TOGETHER TO ONE SIDE** and then to the other so your lower body makes a windshield wiper motion. **LET YOUR HIPS ROLL WITH YOUR KNEES.** That's 1 rep. Continue for the prescribed number of reps; repeat with your palms facing up.

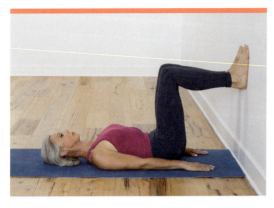

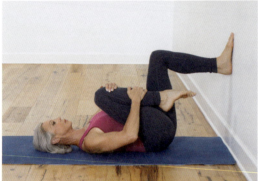

Single-Leg Stretch

SETUP

Lie on a mat and place your feet flat on the wall hip-width apart, knees bent 90 degrees. Place your arms down by your sides. Keep your back long and flat to the mat.

STEPS

1 **BEND YOUR RIGHT KNEE TOWARD YOUR CHEST,** keeping your hip, knee, and ankle aligned. **PLACE YOUR HANDS ON YOUR RIGHT SHIN AND DRAW YOUR RIGHT THIGH** toward your chest so your knee reaches between your shoulder and your ear. (Place your hands under your right thigh if your knee is sensitive.) Hold for the prescribed amount of time. Place your foot back on the wall.

2 Repeat with your right side for the prescribed amount of time.

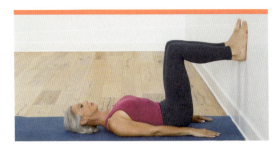

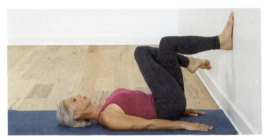

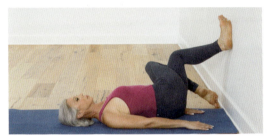

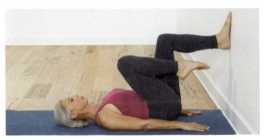

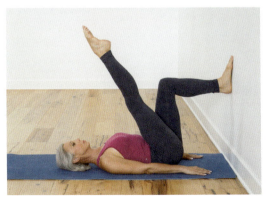

Cross-Leg Twist

SETUP

Lie on a mat and place your feet flat on the wall hip-width apart, knees bent 90 degrees. Place your arms down by your sides. Keep your back long and flat to the mat.

STEPS

1 **BEND YOUR RIGHT KNEE** to your chest and cross it over your left knee.

2 **TWIST TOWARD THE LEFT WHILE** keeping your shoulders flat on the floor. Untwist so your right knee is back at your chest. **EXTEND YOUR RIGHT FOOT TOWARD THE CEILING** and put your foot back on the wall. That's 1 rep. Continue for the prescribed number of reps; then repeat on the left side.

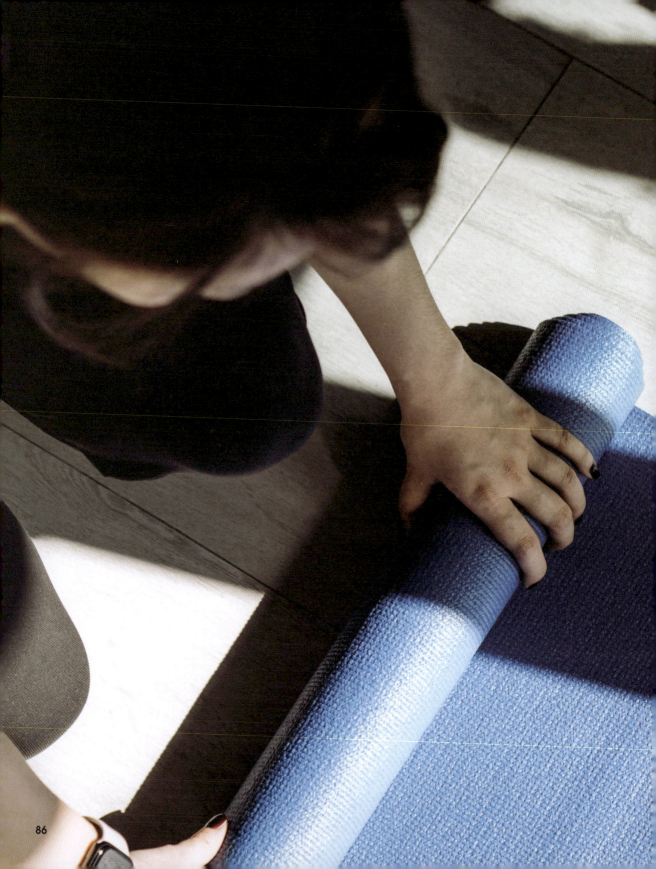

Workout
EXERCISES
▶ P. 88 – 131

The Hundred

The Roll-Up

The One-Leg Circle

The Single-Leg Stretch

The Double-Leg Stretch

The Crisscross

The Spine Stretch Forward

The Teaser Preparation

The One-Leg Kickback

The Side-Kick Series

The Spine Twist

The Hundred

CHECK YOUR FORM

ROLL UP high enough to engage your upper stomach

PUMP your arms vigorously and evenly

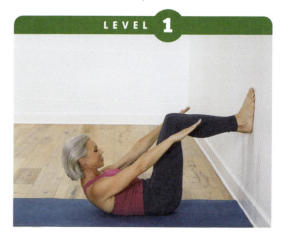

LEVEL 1

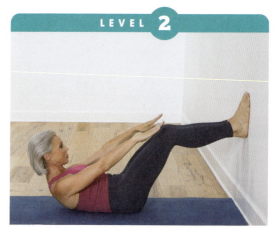

LEVEL 2

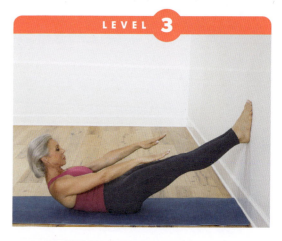

LEVEL 3

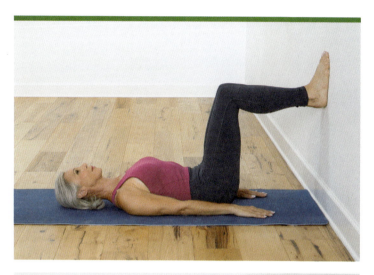

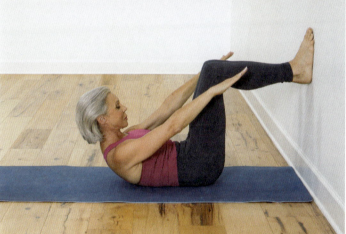

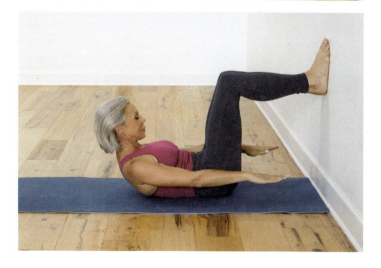

The
Hundred

L E V E L

1

SETUP

Lie on a mat and place your feet on the wall hip-width apart, knees bent 90 degrees. Place your arms down by your sides. Keep your back long and flat to the mat.

STEPS

1 **ROLL YOUR SHOULDERS** off the mat while gazing toward your navel and **KEEPING YOUR CHIN TUCKED** toward your chest.

2 Raise your arms 6 to 8 inches above the mat. **VIGOR-OUSLY PUMP YOUR ARMS UP ONCE AND DOWN ONCE.** That's 1 rep. Continue for the prescribed number of reps while inhaling through your nose for 5 seconds and then exhaling for 5 seconds through your nose or mouth. (If your neck gets tired, lower your head and keep pumping your arms.)

3 **LOWER YOUR HEAD** to the mat and repeat for the prescribed number of reps, while continuing the same breathing pattern.

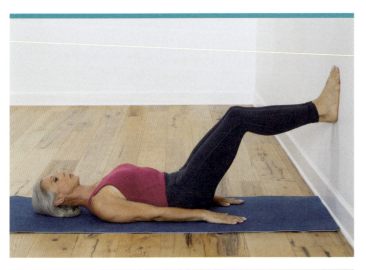

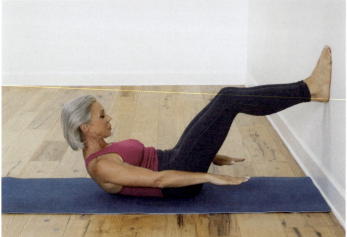

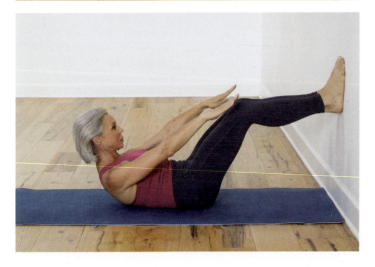

LEVEL
2

Follow the same setup and steps as **THE HUNDRED: LEVEL 1**, but in the setup **bend your knees 45 degrees** instead of 90.

SETUP

Lie on a mat and place your feet on the wall hip-width apart, knees bent 45 degrees. Place your arms down by your sides. Keep your back long and flat to the mat.

STEPS

1 **ROLL YOUR SHOULDERS** off the mat while gazing toward your navel and keeping your chin tucked toward your chest.

2 Raise your arms 6 to 8 inches above the mat. **VIGOR-OUSLY PUMP YOUR ARMS UP ONCE AND DOWN ONCE.** That's 1 rep. Continue for the prescribed number of reps while inhaling through your nose for 5 seconds and then exhaling for 5 seconds through your nose or mouth. (If your neck gets tired, lower your head and keep pumping your arms.)

3 **LOWER YOUR HEAD** to the mat and repeat for the prescribed number of reps, while continuing the same breathing pattern.

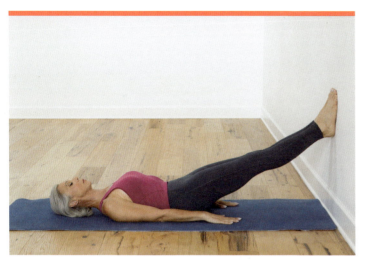

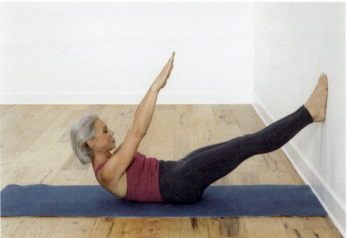

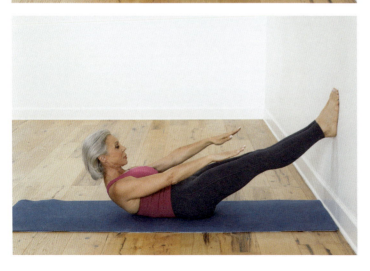

L E V E L
3

Follow the same setup and steps as **THE HUNDRED: LEVEL 1**, but in the setup **lie on a mat with your legs straight and your feet touching the wall** instead of bending your knees 90 degrees.

SETUP

Lie on a mat with your legs straight and feet touching the wall. Place your arms down by your sides. Keep your back long and flat to the mat.

STEPS

1 **ROLL YOUR SHOULDERS** off the mat while gazing toward your navel and keeping your chin tucked toward your chest.

2 Raise your arms 6 to 8 inches above the mat. **VIGOR-OUSLY PUMP YOUR ARMS UP ONCE AND DOWN ONCE.** That's 1 rep. Continue for the prescribed number of reps while inhaling through your nose for 5 seconds and then exhaling for 5 seconds through your nose or mouth. (If your neck gets tired, lower your head and keep pumping your arms.)

3 **LOWER YOUR HEAD** to the mat and repeat for the prescribed number of reps, while continuing the same breathing pattern.

The Roll-Up

CHECK YOUR FORM

DON'T ARCH your neck as your arms reach overhead

DON'T LOCK your elbows

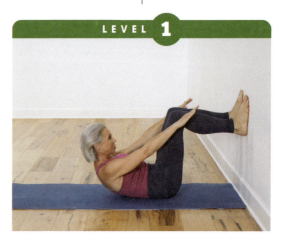

LEVEL 1

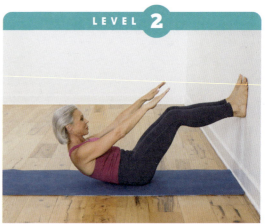

LEVEL 2

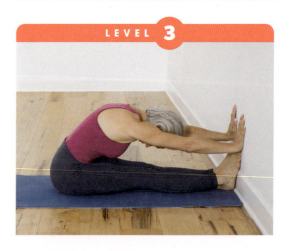

LEVEL 3

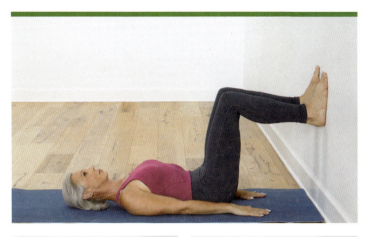

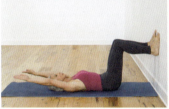
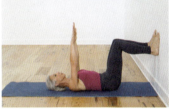

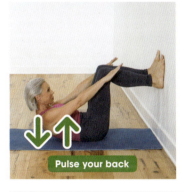

Pulse your back

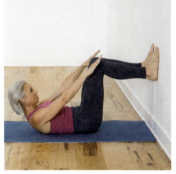

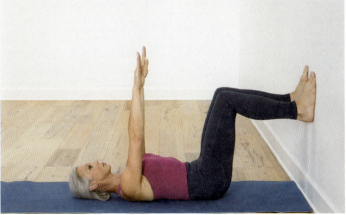

The Roll-Up

L E V E L

1

SETUP

Lie on a mat and place your feet flat on the wall hip-width apart, knees bent 90 degrees. Place your arms down by your sides. Keep your back long and flat to the mat.

STEPS

1 Reach your arms over the top of your head. Inhale and **LIFT YOUR ARMS TO THE CEILING, FOLLOWED BY YOUR HEAD.**

2 **EXHALE AND ROLL YOUR SHOULDERS** off the mat while gazing toward your navel and **KEEPING YOUR CHIN TUCKED** toward your chest. Lower your arms and reach them forward as you roll up. Keep your waist and lower back on the mat.

3 Inhale through your nose and **PULSE YOUR BACK BY LIFTING YOUR WAIST UP** off the mat (like you're doing a sit-up) then lowering back down. That's 1 rep. Continue pulsing for the prescribed number of reps, inhaling for 5 seconds and exhaling through your nose or mouth for 5 seconds.

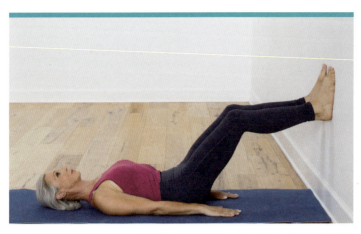

Follow the same setup
and steps as **THE ROLL-UP:
LEVEL 1**, but in the setup
**bend your knees 45
degrees instead of 90**.

SETUP

Lie on a mat and place your feet flat
on the wall hip-width apart, knees
bent 45 degrees. Place your arms
down by your sides. Keep your back
long and flat to the mat.

STEPS

1 Reach your arms over the top
of your head. Inhale and **LIFT
YOUR ARMS TO THE
CEILING, FOLLOWED BY
YOUR HEAD.**

2 **EXHALE AND ROLL YOUR
SHOULDERS** off the mat
while gazing toward your navel
and **KEEPING YOUR CHIN
TUCKED** toward your chest.
Lower your arms and reach
them forward as you roll up.
Keep your waist and lower back
on the mat.

3 Inhale through your nose and
**PULSE YOUR BACK BY
LIFTING YOUR WAIST
UP OFF THE MAT** (like
you're doing a sit-up) then
lowering back down. That's 1
rep. Continue pulsing for the
prescribed number of reps,
inhaling for 5 seconds and
exhaling through your nose or
mouth for 5 seconds.

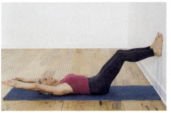

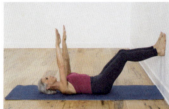

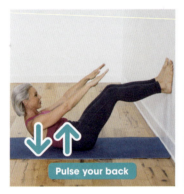

Pulse your back

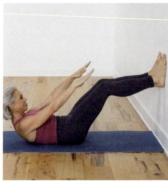

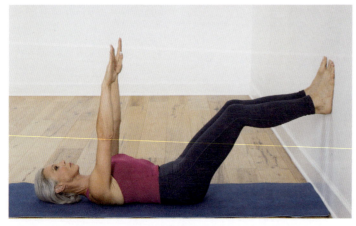

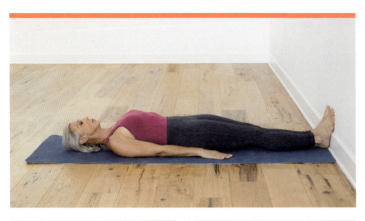

LEVEL
3

SETUP

Lie on a mat with your feet touching the wall. Place your arms down by your sides. Keep your back long and flat to the mat.

STEPS

1 Reach your arms over the top of your head. Inhale and **LIFT YOUR ARMS TO THE CEILING, FOLLOWED BY YOUR HEAD.**

2 **EXHALE AND ROLL YOUR SHOULDERS** off the mat while gazing toward your navel and **KEEPING YOUR CHIN TUCKED** toward your chest. Lower your arms and reach them forward as you roll up, reaching your forehead toward your knees. As you reach, press your feet on the wall.

3 Inhale and roll back down to the mat. **EXHALE WHILE LIFTING YOUR ARMS UP TOWARD THE CEILING AND BACK OVER THE TOP OF YOUR HEAD.** That's 1 rep. Continue for the prescribed number of reps.

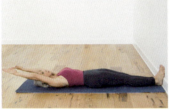
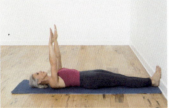
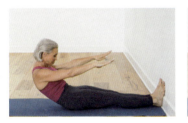
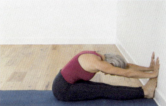
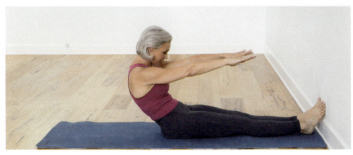
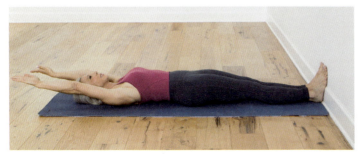

The One-Leg Circle

CHECK YOUR FORM

AVOID ROCKING your pelvis, hips, or shoulders

STRAIGHTEN your lifted leg as much as you can without locking your knee

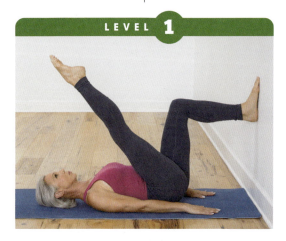

LEVEL 1

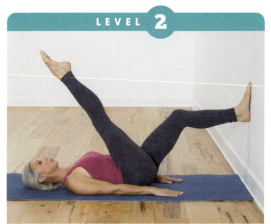

LEVEL 2

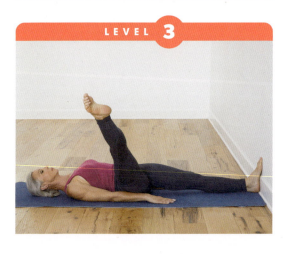

LEVEL 3

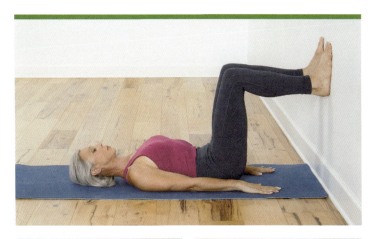

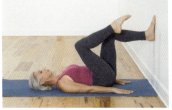
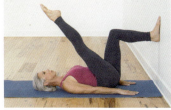

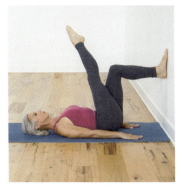
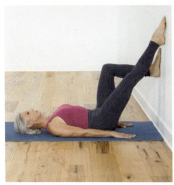

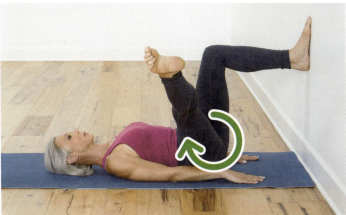

The One-Leg Circle

LEVEL
1

SETUP

Lie on a mat and place your feet flat on the wall hip-width apart, knees bent 90 degrees. Place your arms down by your sides. Keep your back long and flat to the mat.

STEPS

1 **INHALE WHILE BENDING** your right leg toward your chest, keeping your leg in line with your hip. Exhale, point your right foot, and extend it toward the ceiling.

2 **INHALE AND BRING** your right leg toward your nose.

3 **EXHALE** as you cross your right leg slightly to the left. Hold for 3 seconds.

4 **INHALE AND LOWER** your leg toward the wall. Hold for 3 seconds.

5 **EXHALE AND OPEN** your leg slightly to the right. Hold for 3 seconds.

6 Repeat steps 2 through 5 to make 4 more small clockwise circles. Reverse the motion and make 5 counterclockwise circles.

7 **BEND** your right leg to your chest and put your foot back on the wall. That's 1 rep. Continue for the prescribed number of reps; repeat with your left leg.

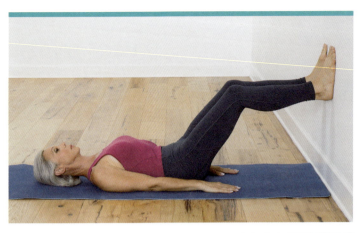

Follow the same setup and steps as **THE ONE-LEG CIRCLE: LEVEL 1**, but in the setup **bend your knees 45 degrees** instead of 90.

SETUP

Lie on a mat with your feet hip-width on the wall, knees bent 45 degrees, arms by your sides, and back long and flat to the mat.

STEPS

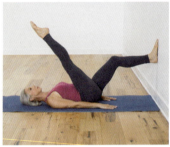

1 **INHALE WHILE BENDING** your right leg in toward your chest. Exhale, point your right foot, and extend it toward the ceiling.

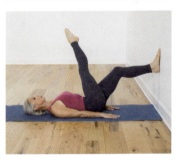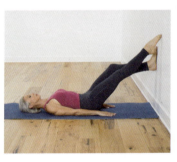

2 **INHALE AND BRING** your right leg toward your nose. Hold for 3 seconds.

3 **EXHALE** as you cross your right leg slightly toward the left. Hold for 3 seconds.

4 **INHALE AND LOWER** your leg toward the center, hovering your foot near the wall. Hold for 3 seconds.

5 **EXHALE AND OPEN** your leg slightly to the right. Hold for 3 seconds.

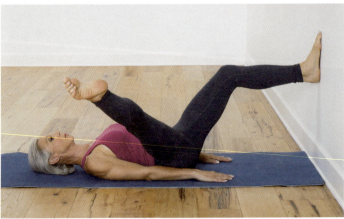

6 Repeat steps 2 through 5 to make 4 more small counter-clockwise circles. Reverse the motion and make 5 clockwise circles.

7 **BEND** your right leg to your chest and put your foot back on the wall. That's 1 rep. Continue for the prescribed number of reps; repeat with your left leg.

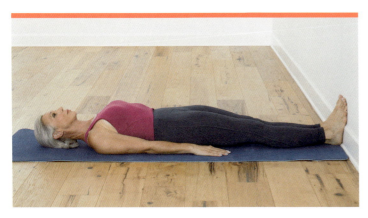

Follow the same setup and steps as **THE ONE-LEG CIRCLE: LEVEL 1**, but in the setup **lie with your legs straight** instead of bending your knees.

SETUP

Lie on a mat with your legs straight, feet on the wall, arms by your sides, and back long and flat to the mat.

STEPS

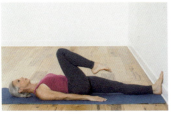
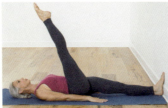
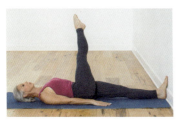
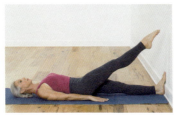

1 **INHALE WHILE BENDING** your right leg in toward your chest. Exhale, point your right foot, and extend it toward the ceiling.

2 **INHALE AND BRING** your right leg toward your nose. Hold for 3 seconds.

3 **EXHALE** as you cross your right leg slightly toward the left. Hold for 3 seconds.

4 **INHALE AND LOWER** your leg toward the center, your foot near the wall. Hold for 3 seconds.

5 **EXHALE AND OPEN** your leg slightly to the right. Hold for 3 seconds.

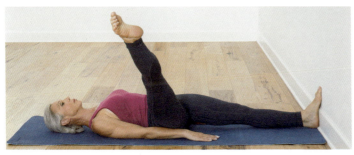

6 Repeat steps 2 through 5 to make 4 more small counterclockwise circles. Reverse the motion and make 5 clockwise circles.

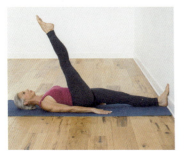
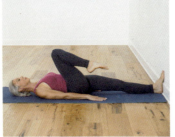

7 **BEND** your right leg to your chest and put your foot back on the wall. That's 1 rep. Continue for the prescribed number of reps; repeat with your left leg.

The Single-Leg Stretch

CHECK YOUR FORM

AVOID ROLLING to one side when lifting or lowering your pelvis

KEEP YOUR HIPS centered when pressing your leg to your chest

AT-A-GLANCE

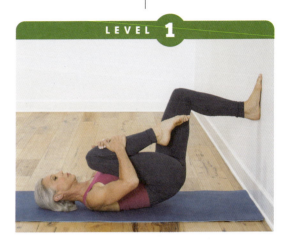

LEVEL **1**

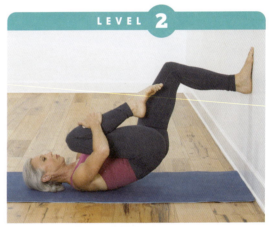

LEVEL **2**

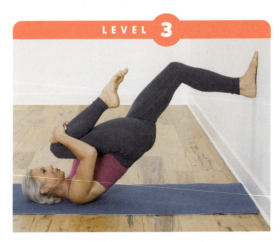

LEVEL **3**

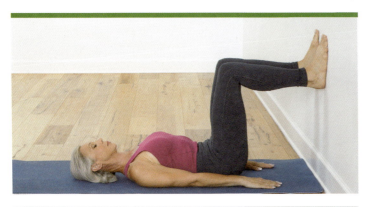

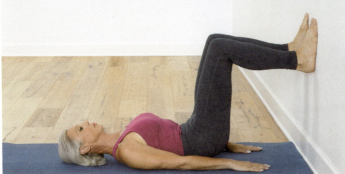

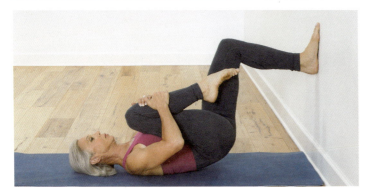

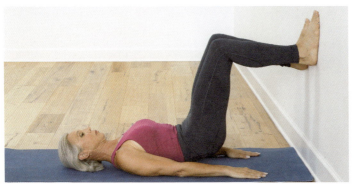

The Single-Leg Stretch

LEVEL

1

SETUP

Lie on a mat and place your feet flat on the wall hip-width apart, knees bent 90 degrees. Place your arms down by your sides. Keep your back long and flat to the mat.

STEPS

1 **INHALE FULLY,** then exhale and tip your tailbone up to lift it off the mat.

2 **INHALE FULLY,** then exhale while bringing your right knee into your chest. Hold your right shin with your hands and press your leg into your chest for 3 seconds.

3 **INHALE AND RETURN** your right foot to the wall. Lower your tailbone down to the mat. That's 1 rep.

4 **REPEAT** with your left leg. Continue alternating for the prescribed number of reps.

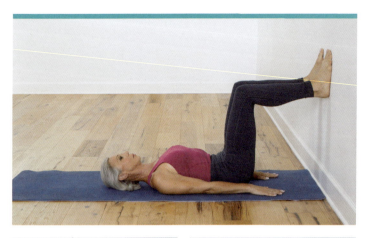

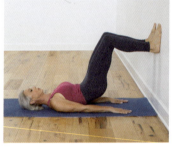
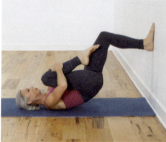

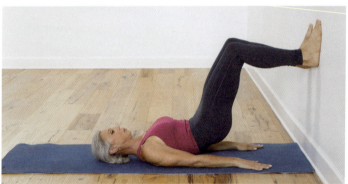

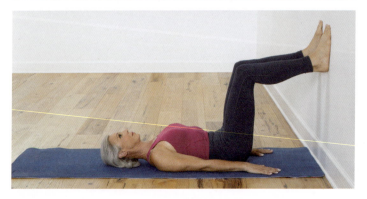

The Single-Leg Stretch
LEVEL
2

Follow the same setup and steps as **THE SINGLE-LEG STRETCH: LEVEL 1**, but in Step 1 **lift your tailbone and pelvis—stopping at your waist**—instead of only your tailbone.

SETUP

Lie on a mat and place your feet flat on the wall hip-width apart, knees bent 90 degrees. Place your arms down by your sides. Keep your back long and flat to the mat.

STEPS

1 **INHALE FULLY,** then exhale and tip your tailbone up to lift your pelvis off the mat.

2 **INHALE FULLY,** then exhale while bringing your right knee into your chest. Hold your right shin with your hands and press your leg into your chest for 3 seconds.

3 **INHALE AND RETURN** your right foot to the wall. Lower your tailbone down to the mat. That's 1 rep.

4 **REPEAT** with your left leg. Continue alternating for the prescribed amount of reps.

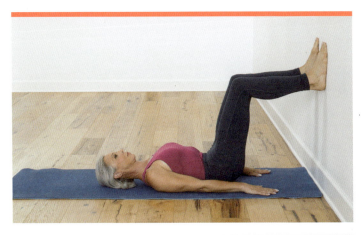

Follow the same setup and steps as **THE SINGLE-LEG STRETCH: LEVEL 1**, but in Step 1 **lift your tail-bone, pelvis, and ribs** instead of only your tailbone.

SETUP

Lie on a mat and place your feet flat on the wall hip-width apart, knees bent 90 degrees. Place your arms down by your sides. Keep your back long and flat to the mat.

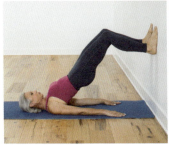
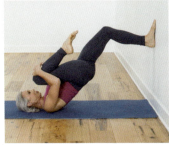

STEPS

1 **INHALE FULLY,** then exhale and tip your tailbone up to lift your pelvis, waist, and ribs off the mat.

2 **INHALE FULLY,** then exhale while bringing your right knee into your chest. Hold your right shin with your hands and press your leg into your chest for 3 seconds.

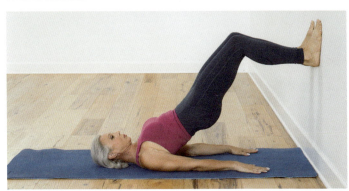

3 **INHALE AND RETURN** your right foot to the wall Lower your tailbone down to the mat. That's 1 rep.

4 **REPEAT** with your left leg. Continue alternating for the prescribed amount of reps.

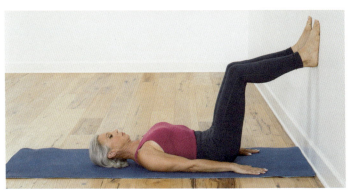

The Double-Leg Stretch

CHECK YOUR FORM

STAY CENTERED when lifting or lowering your pelvis

AVOID ARCHING your back

LEAVE YOUR ARMS by your sides if the overhead arm position is too difficult

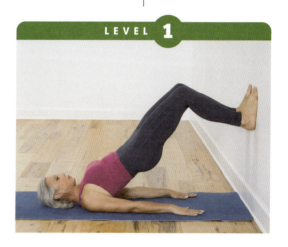

LEVEL 1

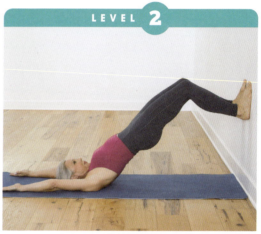

LEVEL 2

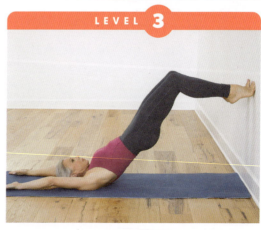

LEVEL 3

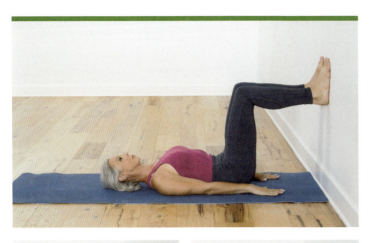

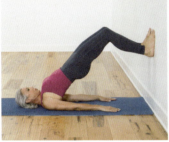
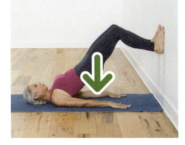

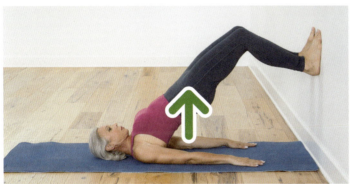

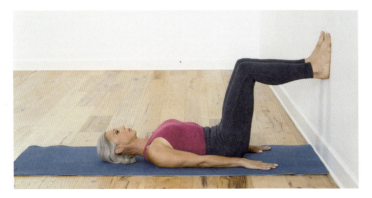

The Double-Leg Stretch

L E V E L

1

S E T U P

Lie on a mat and place your feet flat on the wall hip-width apart, knees bent 90 degrees. Place your arms down by your sides. Keep your back long and flat to the mat.

S T E P S

1 **INHALE FULLY,** then exhale and tip your tailbone up to lift your pelvis, waist, and ribs off the mat. Stop lifting at your shoulders.

2 **INHALE** as you pulse your pelvis up and down for 5 seconds, pressing into the soles of your feet as you pulse.

3 **EXHALE** as you gradually roll your ribs, waist, and pelvis back down to the mat. That's 1 rep. Continue for the prescribed number of reps.

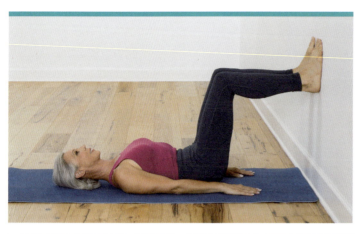

The Double-Leg Stretch

LEVEL

2

SETUP

Lie on a mat and place your feet flat on the wall hip-width apart, knees bent 90 degrees. Place your arms down by your sides. Keep your back long and flat to the mat.

STEPS

1 **INHALE DEEPLY AND LIFT** your arms toward the ceiling and back overhead as far as you can comfortably reach.

2 **EXHALE AND TIP** your tailbone up to lift your pelvis, waist, and ribs off the mat. Stop lifting at your shoulders.

3 **INHALE AS YOU PULSE** your pelvis up and down for 10 seconds, pressing into the soles of your feet as you pulse.

4 **EXHALE AS YOU GRAD-UALLY ROLL** your ribs, waist, and pelvis back down to the mat. Bring your arms back down to your sides. That's 1 rep. Continue for the prescribed number of reps.

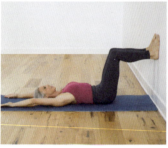
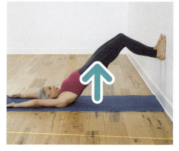
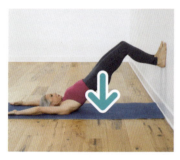
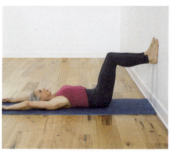
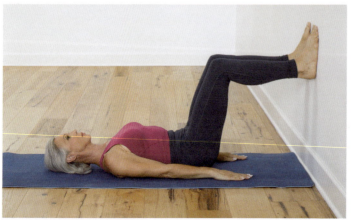

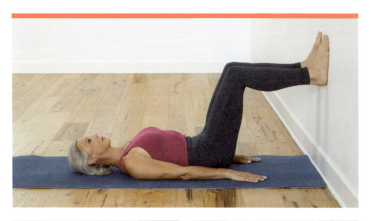

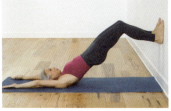
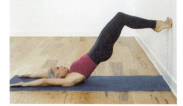

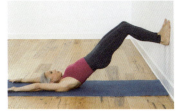
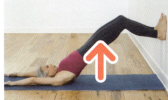

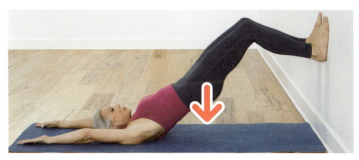

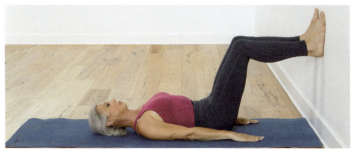

The Double-Leg Stretch
LEVEL
3

Follow the same setup and steps as **THE DOUBLE-LEG STRETCH: LEVEL 2,** but **lift and lower your heels 5 times** in Step 3. Then, in Step 4, pulse your pelvis up and down for 15 seconds instead of 10.

SETUP

Lie on a mat and place your feet flat on the wall hip-width apart, knees bent 90 degrees. Place your arms down by your sides. Keep your back long and flat to the mat.

STEPS

1 **INHALE DEEPLY AND LIFT** your arms toward the ceiling and back overhead as far as you can comfortably reach.

2 **EXHALE AND TIP** your tailbone up to lift your pelvis, waist, and ribs off the mat. Stop lifting at your shoulders.

3 **LIFT AND LOWER** your heels 5 times.

4 **INHALE AS YOU PULSE** your pelvis up and down for 15 seconds, pressing into the soles of your feet as you pulse.

5 **EXHALE AS YOU GRAD-UALLY ROLL** your ribs, waist, and pelvis back down to the mat. Bring your arms back down to your sides. That's 1 rep. Continue for the prescribed number of reps.

The Crisscross

CHECK YOUR FORM

DON'T ROLL to one side as you twist

KEEP YOUR FEET pressing into the wall

ANCHOR YOUR PELVIS as you twist

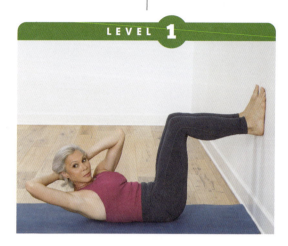

LEVEL 1

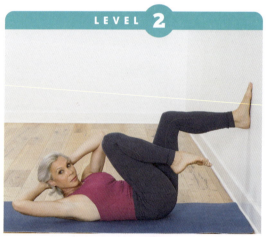

LEVEL 2

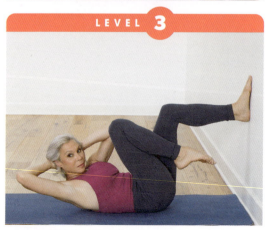

LEVEL 3

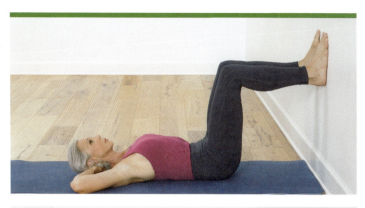

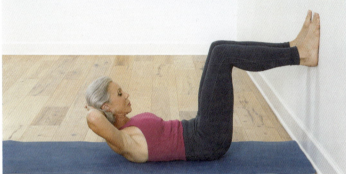

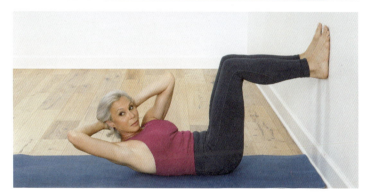

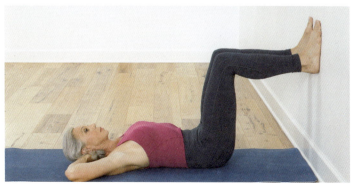

L E V E L
1

SETUP

Lie on a mat and place your feet flat on the wall hip-width apart, knees bent 90 degrees. Place your hands behind your head like you would to do a sit-up. Keep your back long and flat to the mat.

STEPS

1 Inhale deeply. **EXHALE AND ROLL** your shoulders off the mat, tucking your chin to your chest. Keep your elbows open wide as you roll up.

2 **INHALE WHILE PRESS-ING** your feet into the wall.

3 **EXHALE AND TWIST** your left elbow toward your right knee. Your gaze should look past your right elbow.

4 **INHALE DEEPLY AND UNTWIST.** Roll back down to the mat. That's 1 rep. Continue for the prescribed number of reps; repeat on the left side.

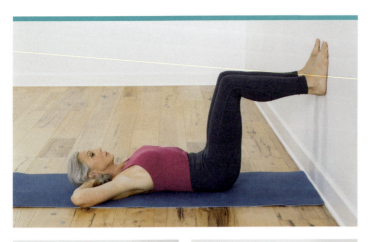

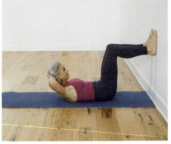

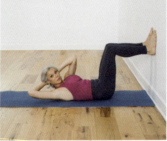

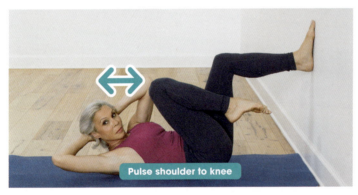

Pulse shoulder to knee

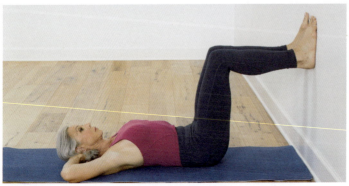

Follow the same setup and steps as **THE CRISSCROSS: LEVEL 1**, but in Step 4 and Step 5 **bend your right knee into your chest and pulse your shoulders** slightly higher for 5 seconds.

SETUP

Lie on a mat and place your feet flat on the wall hip-width apart, knees bent 90 degrees. Place your hands behind your head like you would to do a sit-up. Keep your back long and flat to the mat.

STEPS

1 Inhale deeply. **EXHALE AND ROLL** your shoulders off the mat, tucking your chin to your chest.

2 **INHALE WHILE PRESSING** your feet into the wall.

3 **EXHALE AND TWIST** your left elbow toward your right knee. Your gaze should look past your right elbow.

4 **BEND** your right knee into your chest.

5 **PULSE** your shoulder slightly higher than Level 1 for 5 seconds.

6 Place your right foot back on the wall. Return to center and look toward your navel. Roll back down to the mat. That's 1 rep. Continue for the prescribed number of reps; repeat on the left side.

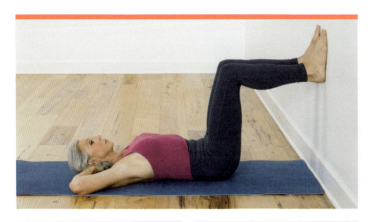

Follow the same setup and steps as **THE CRISSCROSS: LEVEL 2,** but after placing your right foot back on the wall and untwisting, **twist to the right again and pulse your shoulders** slightly higher for 5 seconds.

SETUP

Lie on a mat and place your feet flat on the wall hip-width apart, knees bent 90 degrees. Place your hands behind your head. Keep your back long and flat to the mat.

STEPS

1 Inhale deeply. **EXHALE AND ROLL** your shoulders off the mat, tucking your chin.

2 **INHALE WHILE PRESSING** your feet into the wall.

3 **EXHALE AND TWIST** your left elbow toward your right knee. Gaze past your right elbow and bend your right knee to your chest.

4 **PULSE** your shoulder slightly higher than Level 1 for 5 seconds.

5 Place your right foot back on the wall. Return to center and look toward your navel.

6 Repeat steps 3-5, pulsing even higher for 5 seconds.

7 Place your right foot back on the wall, return to center, and roll back. That's 1 rep. Continue for the prescribed number of reps; repeat on the left side.

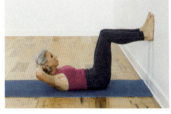

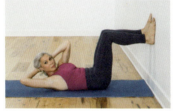

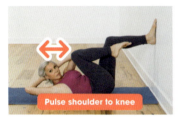

Pulse shoulder to knee

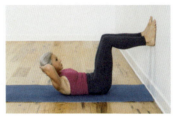

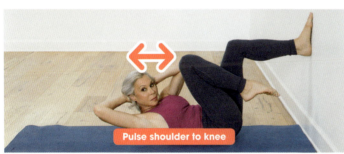

Pulse shoulder to knee

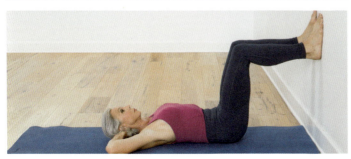

The Spine Stretch Forward

CHECK YOUR FORM

DON'T ROLL your knees in or out

KEEP your shoulders over your hips when seated upright

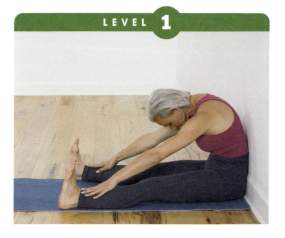

LEVEL 1

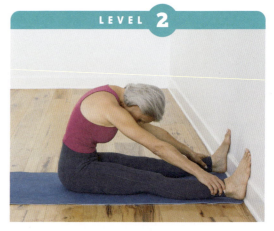

LEVEL 2

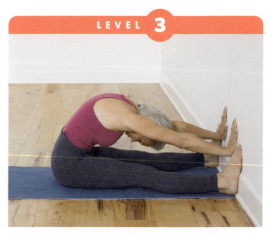

LEVEL 3

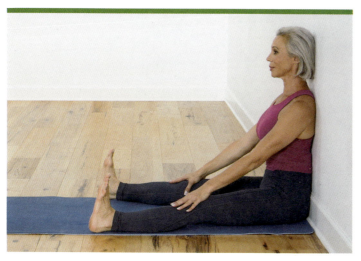

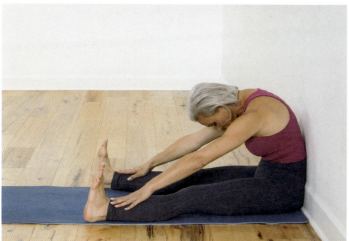

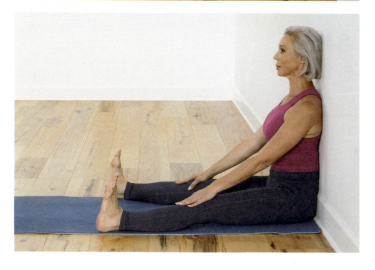

The
Spine Stretch Forward

LEVEL
1

SETUP

Sit upright on the mat with your back against the wall and your legs open slightly wider than your hips. Place your hands on your legs.

STEPS

1 **INHALE DEEPLY AND LOWER** your chin toward your chest. **EXHALE AND PEEL YOUR SHOULDERS AND RIBS OFF THE WALL** while gazing toward your navel. Keep your waist and lower back on the wall. Slide your hands toward your ankles as you round forward. **GRASP YOUR ANKLES IF POSSIBLE,** lifting your stomach as you reach further forward.

2 **EXHALE AND RETURN TO AN UPRIGHT POSITION,** sliding your hands along your legs and rolling your spine back up along the wall. That's 1 rep. Continue for the prescribed number of reps.

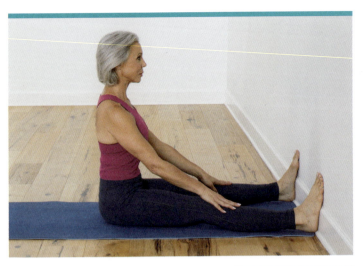

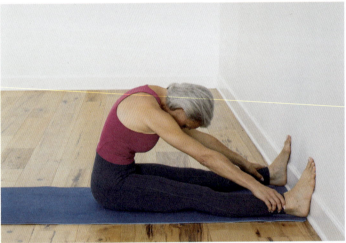

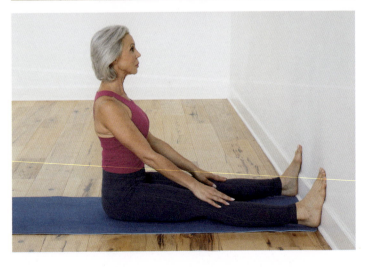

Follow the same setup and steps as **THE SPINE STRETCH FORWARD: LEVEL 1**, but in the setup **sit facing the wall with your feet pressed against the wall** instead of with your back against it.

SETUP

Sit upright on the mat with your feet pressed against the wall and your legs open slightly wider than your hips. Place your hands on your legs.

STEPS

1 **INHALE DEEPLY AND LOWER** your chin toward your chest. **EXHALE AND ROUND YOUR SHOULDERS AND RIBS FORWARD** while gazing toward your navel. **SLIDE YOUR HANDS TOWARD** your ankles as you round forward. Grasp your ankles if possible, lifting your stomach as you reach further forward.

2 **EXHALE AND RETURN** to an upright position, **SLIDING YOUR HANDS** along your legs and rolling your spine back up. That's 1 rep. Continue for the prescribed number of reps.

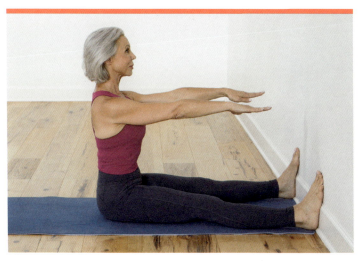

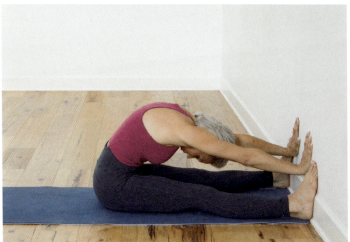

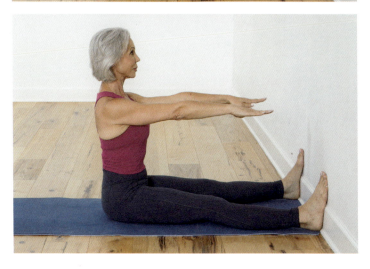

The
Spine Stretch Forward

LEVEL
3

Follow the same setup and steps as **THE SPINE STRETCH FORWARD: LEVEL 2**, but in the setup **extend your arms forward at shoulder height instead of placing your hands on your legs.**

SETUP

Sit upright on the mat with your feet pressed against the wall and your legs open slightly wider than your hips. Extend your arms forward at shoulder height.

STEPS

1 Inhale deeply and **LOWER YOUR CHIN** toward your chest. Exhale and **ROUND YOUR SHOULDERS AND RIBS FORWARD** while gazing toward your navel. Reach your hands forward, touching the wall if possible while lifting your stomach.

2 Exhale and **RETURN TO AN UPRIGHT POSITION.** That's 1 rep. Continue for the prescribed number of reps.

The Teaser Preparation

CHECK YOUR FORM

DON'T ROLL your knees in or out

AVOID LOCKING your elbows when your arms are overhead

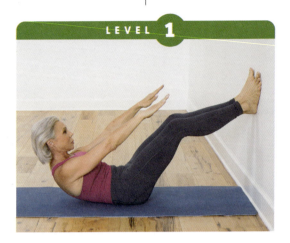

LEVEL 1

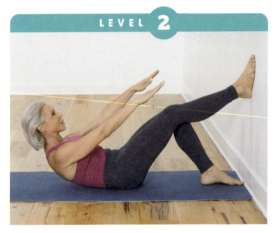

LEVEL 2

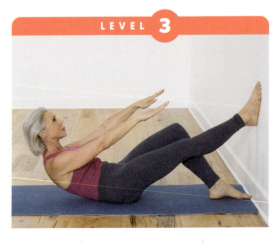

LEVEL 3

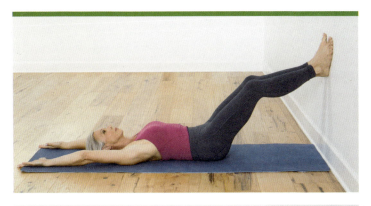

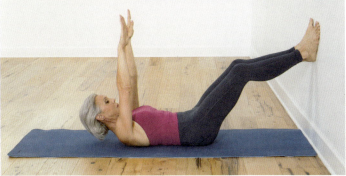

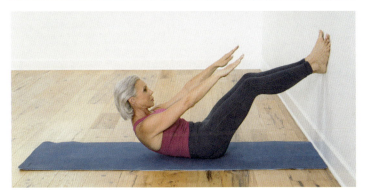

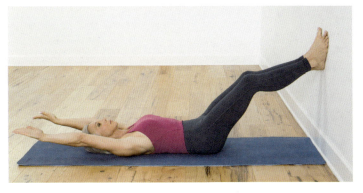

The
Teaser Preparation

LEVEL
1

SETUP

Lie on a mat and place your feet flat on the wall with heels together and toes and knees apart, knees bent 45 degrees. Reach your arms over the top of your head.

STEPS

1 Inhale and **LIFT YOUR ARMS TOWARD THE CEILING WHILE PRESSING YOUR SHOULDERS** into the mat. Continue inhaling and lift your head.

2 Exhale and roll your shoulders off the mat as you **LOWER YOUR ARMS TO REACH FORWARD AND TUCK YOUR CHIN TO YOUR CHEST.** Keep your lower back on the mat.

3 Inhale through your nose. Exhale through your nose or mouth and **ROLL BACK DOWN TO THE MAT, BRINGING YOUR ARMS BACK OVERHEAD.** That's 1 rep. Continue for the prescribed number of reps.

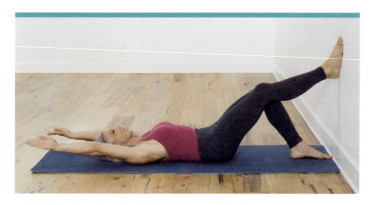

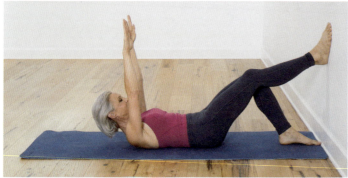

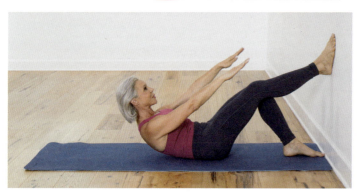

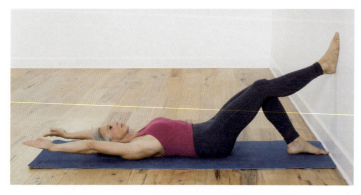

Follow the same setup and steps as **THE TEASER PREPARATION: LEVEL 1**, but in the setup **bend your left leg and place your left foot** on the floor instead of keeping both feet on the wall.

SETUP

Lie on a mat and place your right foot flat on the wall, knee bent 45 degrees, and your left foot on the mat, knee bent. Reach your arms over the top of your head.

STEPS

1 Inhale and **LIFT YOUR ARMS TOWARD THE CEILING WHILE PRESSING YOUR SHOULDERS** into the mat. Continue inhaling and lift your head.

2 Exhale and **ROLL YOUR SHOULDERS** off the mat as you lower your arms to **REACH FORWARD AND TUCK YOUR CHIN** to your chest. Keep your lower back on the mat.

3 Inhale through your nose. Exhale through your nose or mouth and **ROLL BACK DOWN TO THE MAT, BRINGING YOUR ARMS BACK OVERHEAD.** That's 1 rep. Continue for the prescribed number of reps; repeat on the other side.

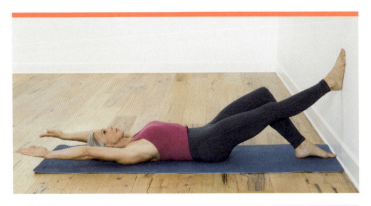

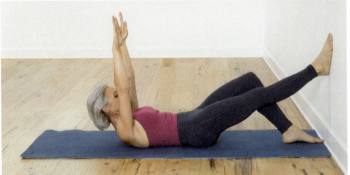

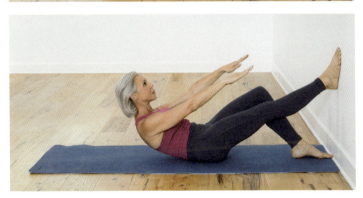

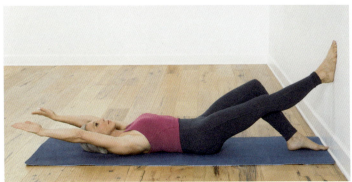

L E V E L
3

Follow the same setup and steps as **THE TEASER PREPARATION: LEVEL 2,** but in the setup **lie with your right foot on the wall, knee straight** instead of bent.

SETUP

Lie on a mat and place your right foot flat on the wall, knee straight, and your left foot on the mat, knee bent. Reach your arms over the top of your head.

STEPS

1 Inhale and **LIFT YOUR ARMS TOWARD THE CEILING WHILE PRESS-ING YOUR SHOULDERS** into the mat. Continue inhaling and lift your head.

2 Exhale and **ROLL YOUR SHOULDERS OFF THE MAT** as you **LOWER YOUR ARMS TO REACH FOR-WARD** and tuck your chin to your chest. Keep your lower back on the mat.

3 Inhale through your nose. Exhale through your nose or mouth and **ROLL BACK DOWN TO THE MAT, BRINGING YOUR ARMS BACK OVERHEAD.** That's 1 rep. Continue for the prescribed number of reps; repeat on the other side.

The One-Leg Kickback

CHECK YOUR FORM

AVOID DROPPING your hip when your leg lowers

KEEP your foot pressing into the wall

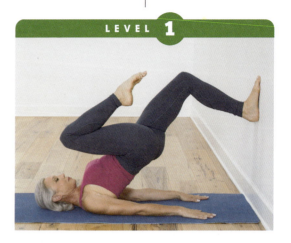

LEVEL 1

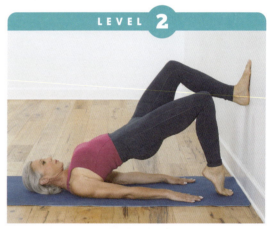

LEVEL 2

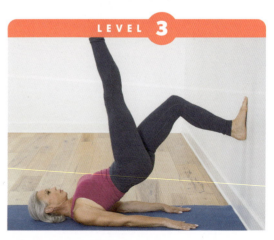

LEVEL 3

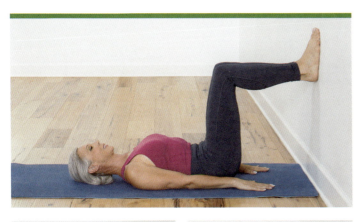

The One-Leg Kickback

L E V E L
1

SETUP

Lie on a mat and place your feet flat on the wall. Your feet should be together and knees bent 90 degrees. Put your arms down by your sides. Keep your back long and flat to the mat.

STEPS

1 Inhale deeply. **EXHALE AND TIP YOUR TAILBONE UP TO LIFT YOUR PELVIS, WAIST, AND RIBS** off the mat, stopping at your shoulders. Avoid putting weight on your neck.

2 Inhale and **BEND YOUR RIGHT KNEE INTO YOUR CHEST.** Tap your right foot down to the mat, keeping it in line with your knee and sit bone, then return it to your chest, then to the wall.

3 Exhale while **ROLLING YOUR RIBS, WAIST, AND PELVIS BACK DOWN TO THE MAT.** That's 1 rep. Continue for the prescribed number of reps; repeat on the left side.

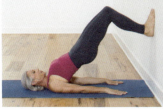
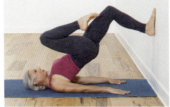
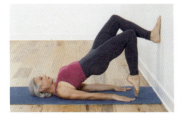
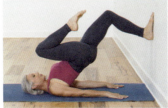
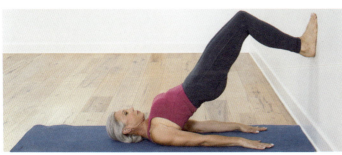
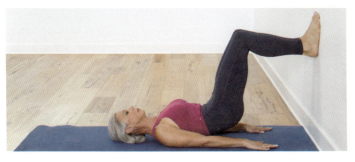

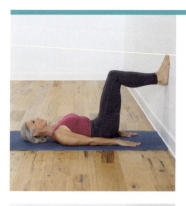
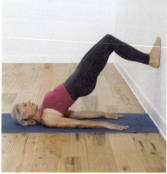
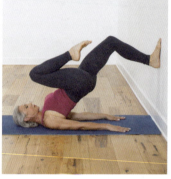
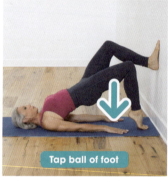

Tap ball of foot

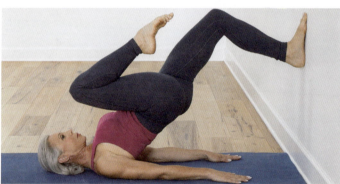

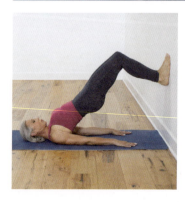
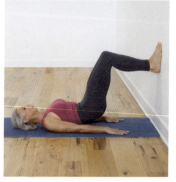

The One-Leg Kickback

LEVEL

2

Follow the same setup and steps as **THE ONE-LEG KICK-BACK: LEVEL 1**, but in Step 2 **tap the ball of your right foot on the floor 5 times** before returning your right knee to your chest.

SETUP

Lie on a mat and place your feet flat on the wall. Your feet should be together and knees bent 90 degrees. Put your arms down by your sides. Keep your back long and flat to the mat.

STEPS

1 Inhale deeply. **EXHALE AND TIP YOUR TAILBONE UP TO LIFT YOUR PELVIS, WAIST, AND RIBS** off the mat, stopping at your shoulders. Avoid putting weight on your neck.

2 Inhale and bend your right knee into your chest. **TAP THE BALL OF YOUR RIGHT FOOT DOWN TO THE MAT 5 TIMES,** keeping it in line with your knee and sit bone, then return it to your chest, then to the wall.

3 Exhale while **ROLLING YOUR RIBS, WAIST, AND PELVIS BACK DOWN TO THE MAT.** That's 1 rep. Continue for the prescribed number of reps; repeat on the left side.

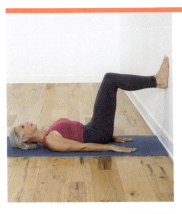
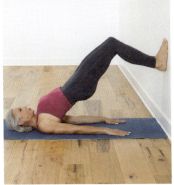
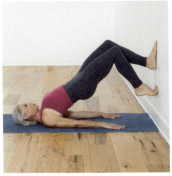
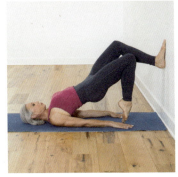
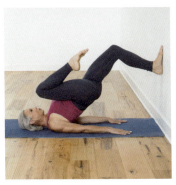
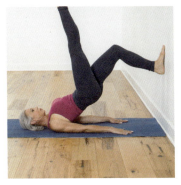
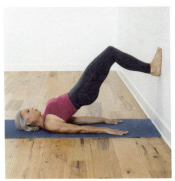
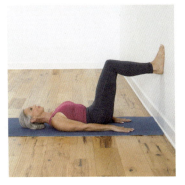

The One-Leg Kickback

L E V E L

3

SETUP

Lie on a mat and place your feet flat on the wall. Keep your feet together, knees bent 90 degrees, and arms down by your sides. Your back should be long and flat to the mat.

STEPS

1 Inhale deeply. **EXHALE AND TIP YOUR TAILBONE UP TO LIFT YOUR PELVIS, WAIST, AND RIBS** off the mat, stopping at your shoulders. Avoid putting weight on your neck.

2 Inhale, **BEND YOUR RIGHT KNEE, AND SLIDE YOUR FOOT DOWN THE WALL TO THE MAT,** keeping your knee and foot in line with your sit bone.

3 Bend your right knee into your chest. **EXTEND THAT LEG; POINT YOUR FOOT AND REACH IT TO THE CEILING.** Return your foot to the wall.

4 Exhale while **ROLLING YOUR RIBS, WAIST, AND PELVIS BACK DOWN TO THE MAT.** That's 1 rep. Continue for the prescribed number of reps; repeat on the left side.

The Side-Kick Series

CHECK YOUR FORM

KEEP your neck long and in line with your spine

AVOID arching your back

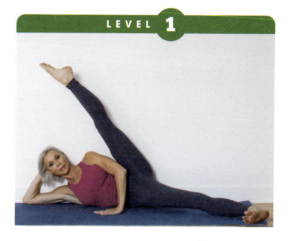

LEVEL 1

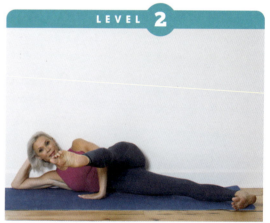

LEVEL 2

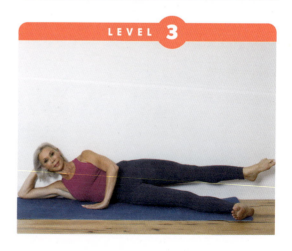

LEVEL 3

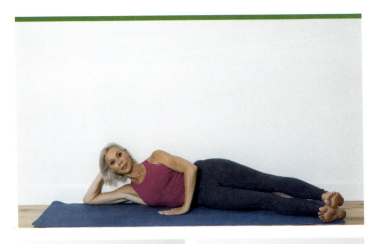

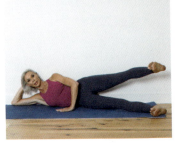 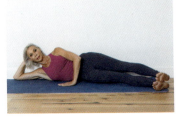

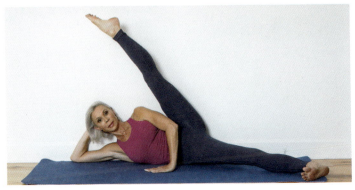

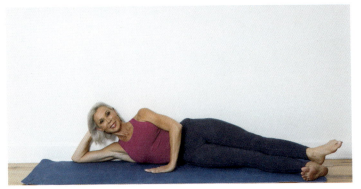

L E V E L

1

S E T U P

Lie on your right side with your back to the wall, legs slightly away from the wall, together and straight. Use your right hand to cradle your head.

S T E P S

1 Inhale deeply while **LIFTING YOUR LEFT LEG SLIGHTLY HIGHER THAN YOUR HIP.** Exhale and press your left leg down, as if squeezing a ball between your legs. Do this 8 times.

2 Rotate your left knee to the ceiling. **KICK YOUR LEFT LEG UP AND IN LINE WITH YOUR LOWER LEG. FLEX YOUR LEFT FOOT AND LOWER YOUR LEG DOWN WITH RESISTANCE.** Do this 8 times. That's 1 rep. Continue for the prescribed number of reps; repeat on the other side.

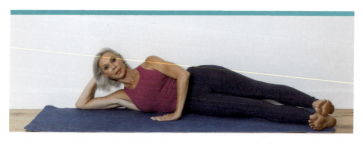

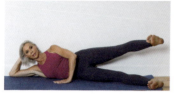
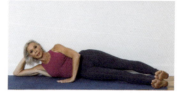

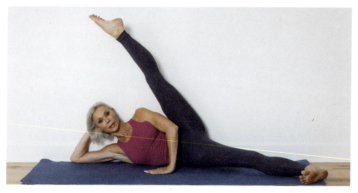

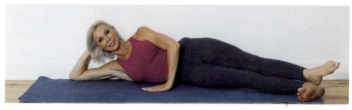

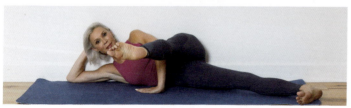

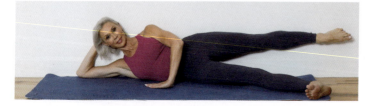

Follow the same setup and steps as **THE SIDE-KICK SERIES: LEVEL 1,** but in Step 2 raise your left leg to hip height and kick your leg forward and backward 8 times.

SETUP

Lie on your right side with your back to the wall, legs slightly away from the wall, together and straight. Use your right hand to cradle your head.

STEPS

1 Inhale deeply **WHILE LIFTING YOUR LEFT LEG SLIGHTLY HIGHER THAN YOUR HIP.** Exhale and press your left leg down, as if squeezing a ball between your legs. Do this 8 times.

2 **ROTATE YOUR LEFT KNEE TO THE CEILING AND KICK YOUR LEFT LEG STRAIGHT UP.** Flex your left foot and lower your leg down with resistance. Do this 8 times.

3 Raise your left leg to hip height. **KICK YOUR LEG FORWARD THEN BACKWARD.** Do this 8 times. That's 1 rep. Continue for the prescribed number of reps; repeat on the other side.

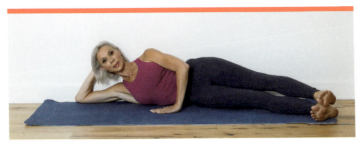

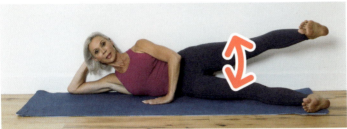

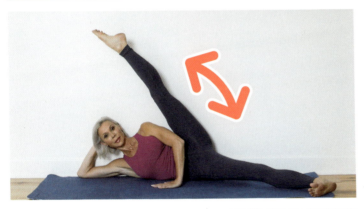

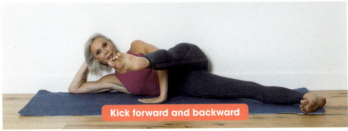

Kick forward and backward

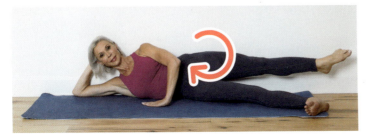

Follow the same setup and steps as **THE SIDE-KICK SERIES: LEVEL 2,** but after kicking your leg forward 8 times, **lower your left leg and make 8 small clockwise circles with it.**

SETUP

Lie on your right side with your back to the wall, legs slightly away from the wall, together and straight. Use your right hand to cradle your head.

STEPS

1 Inhale deeply **WHILE LIFTING YOUR LEFT LEG SLIGHTLY HIGHER THAN YOUR HIP.** Exhale and press your left leg down, as if squeezing a ball between your legs. Do this 8 times.

2 **ROTATE YOUR LEFT KNEE TO THE CEILING AND KICK YOUR LEFT LEG STRAIGHT UP.** Flex your left foot and lower your leg down with resistance. Do this 8 times.

3 Raise your left leg to hip height. **KICK YOUR LEG FORWARD THEN BACKWARD.** Do this 8 times.

4 Lower your left leg. **REACH THE LEG ONE INCH FORWARD AND MAKE A SMALL CLOCKWISE CIRCLE.** Do this 4 times then reverse directions. That's 1 rep. Continue for the prescribed number of reps; repeat on the other side.

The Spine Twist

CHECK YOUR FORM

AVOID ARCHING your lower back

DON'T LOCK your joints

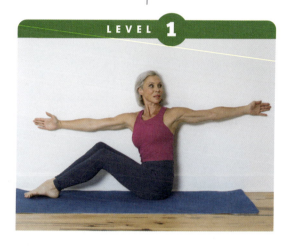

LEVEL 1

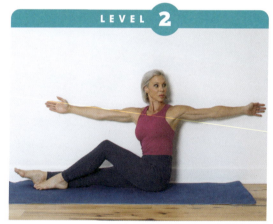

LEVEL 2

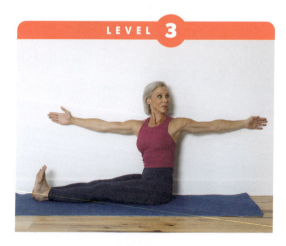

LEVEL 3

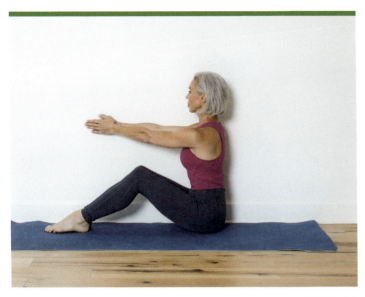

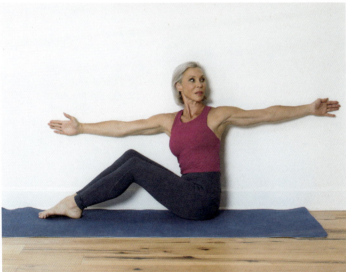

The Spine Twist

LEVEL

1

SETUP

Sit with the right side of your body next to the wall, your knees bent up toward your chest and legs together.

STEPS

1 **REACH YOUR ARMS FORWARD** with palms touching, keeping them at shoulder height. Your right shoulder should be touching the wall. **INHALE AND OPEN YOUR LEFT ARM TO THE SIDE WHILE TURNING YOUR HEAD TO THE LEFT.** Exhale and twist your torso to the left. Reach your hands away from each other to increase the stretch.

2 Inhale and **RETURN TO CENTER WITH YOUR PALMS TOUCHING.** That's 1 rep. Continue for the prescribed number of reps; repeat on the other side.

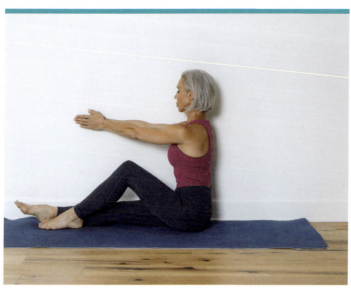

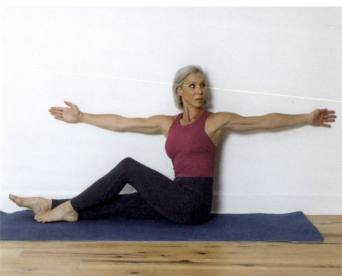

Follow the same setup and steps as **THE SPINE TWIST: LEVEL 1**, but in the setup **sit with your right leg straight** instead of sitting with both legs bent.

SETUP

Sit with the right side of your body next to the wall, your left knee bent up toward your chest, and right leg straight.

STEPS

1 **REACH YOUR ARMS FORWARD** with palms touching, keeping them at shoulder height. Your right shoulder should be touching the wall. Inhale and **OPEN YOUR LEFT ARM TO THE SIDE WHILE TURNING YOUR HEAD TO THE LEFT.** Exhale and twist your torso to the left. Reach your hands away from each other to increase the stretch.

2 Inhale and **RETURN TO CENTER WITH YOUR PALMS TOUCHING.** That's 1 rep. Continue for the prescribed number of reps; repeat on the other side.

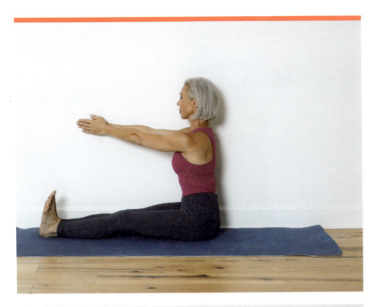

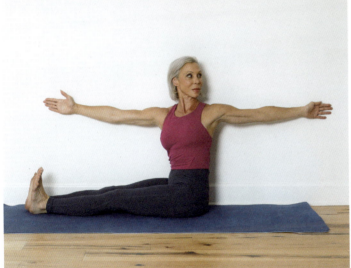

Follow the same setup and
steps as **THE SPINE TWIST:
LEVEL 1**, but in the setup
sit with both legs straight
instead of bent.

SETUP

Sit with the right side of your body
next to the wall, your legs together
and straight.

STEPS

1 **REACH YOUR ARMS
FORWARD** with palms touching, keeping them at shoulder
height. Your right shoulder
should be touching the wall.
Inhale and **OPEN YOUR
LEFT ARM TO THE SIDE
WHILE TURNING YOUR
HEAD TO THE LEFT.**
Exhale and twist your torso to
the left. Reach your hands
away from each other to increase the stretch.

2 Inhale and **RETURN TO
CENTER WITH YOUR
PALMS TOUCHING.**
That's 1 rep. Continue for the
prescribed number of reps;
repeat on the other side.

Cooldown
EXERCISES
▶ **P. 133 – 135**

Roll-Down With Arm Circle
Hug With Elbow Lift
Lying With Legs Up the Wall

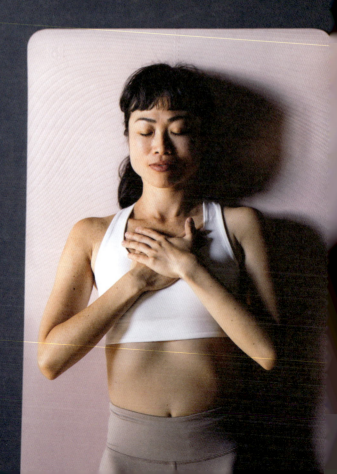

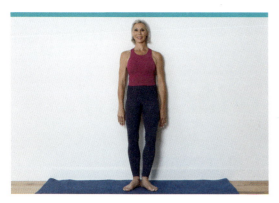

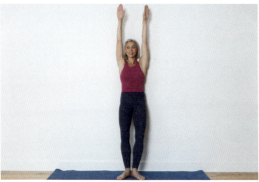

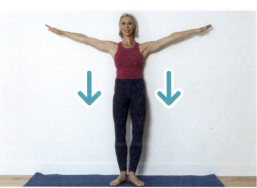

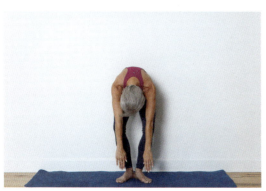

Roll-Down With Arm Circle

CHECK YOUR FORM

KEEP your back long on the wall
AVOID locking your joints

SETUP

Stand with your back leaning against the wall, heels together and about 6 inches from the wall. The balls of your feet should be one hand's-width apart. Soften your knees, lengthen your spine, and place your arms by your sides.

STEPS

1 Inhale deeply and **LIFT YOUR ARMS OVERHEAD** with palms facing forward.

2 Exhale, squeezing all the air out of the lungs as you **LOWER YOUR ARMS TO YOUR SIDES AND FOLD FORWARD** from the waist, tucking your chin into your chest.

3 Inhale, lift your arms forward, and roll your torso up the wall from your waist. **BRING YOUR ARMS OVERHEAD AS THE BACK OF YOUR HEAD RETURNS TO TOUCH THE WALL.** That's 1 rep. Continue for the prescribed number of reps; then repeat, reversing the movement so you start bent over and lift your arms to the sides as you roll up.

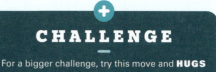

+ CHALLENGE

For a bigger challenge, try this move and **HUGS WITH ELBOW LIFTS** while holding a 1- or 2-pound weight in each hand (or use soup cans).

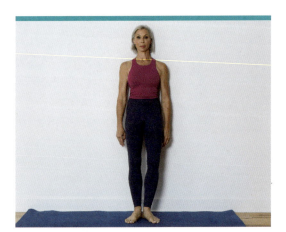

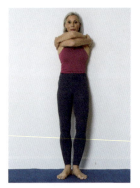
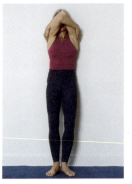

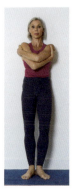
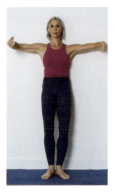
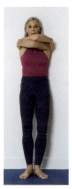

Hug With Elbow Lift

CHECK YOUR FORM

AVOID FLARING your ribs as your elbows lift
KEEP your neck long

SETUP

Stand with your back leaning against the wall, heels together and about 6 inches away from the wall. The balls of your feet should be one hand's-width apart. Soften your knees, lengthen your spine, and place your arms by your sides.

STEPS

1 **CROSS YOUR ARMS OVER YOUR CHEST.** Try to grab as far behind your shoulders as possible.

2 Inhale for 4 seconds **THROUGH THE NOSE WHILE LIFTING YOUR ELBOWS TOWARD YOUR NOSE.** Exhale for 4 seconds and lower your elbows.

3 Inhale and open your arms to the sides. **EXHALE AND CROSS YOUR ARMS OVER YOUR CHEST WITH THE OPPOSITE ARM ON TOP.** That's 1 rep. Continue for the prescribed number of reps; then repeat with the opposite arm on top.

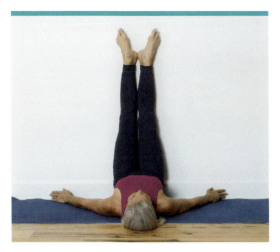

Lying With Legs Up the Wall

SETUP

Lie on a mat with your legs extending up the wall and your bottom as close to the wall as possible.

STEPS

1 Inhale and exhale for **25 SLOW BREATHS.**

2 Bend your knees open to the sides, **PRESSING THE BOTTOMS OF YOUR FEET TOGETHER.**

3 Inhale and place your hands on your thighs. **EXHALE AND PRESS YOUR THIGHS OPEN. INHALE AND RELEASE THE PRESSURE.** That's 1 rep. Continue for prescribed number of reps.

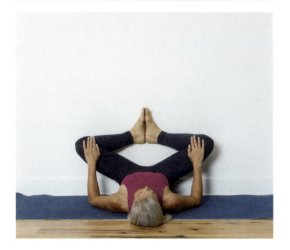

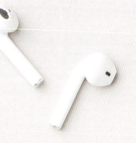

Standing
EXERCISES
▶ P. 137 – 157

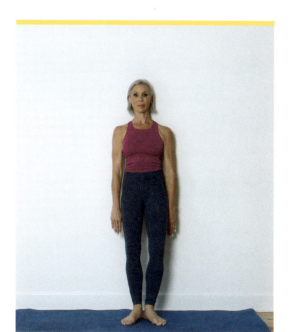

Arm Lower and Lift Front

SETUP

Stand with your back against the wall, your heels together and the balls of your feet slightly apart. Soften your knees and pull your stomach up and in. Place your arms by your sides.

STEPS

1 Inhale and **LIFT YOUR ARMS OVERHEAD** toward the ceiling, palms facing forward.

2 Exhale, **SQUEEZING ALL THE AIR OUT OF YOUR LUNGS WHILE LOWERING YOUR ARMS** back down to your sides. That's 1 rep. Continue for the prescribed number of reps.

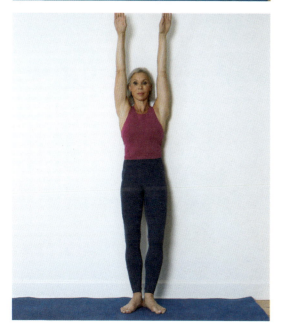

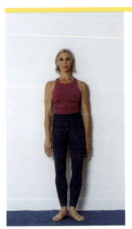
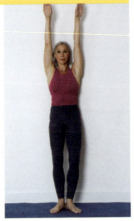
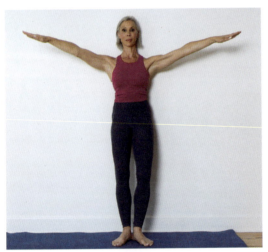
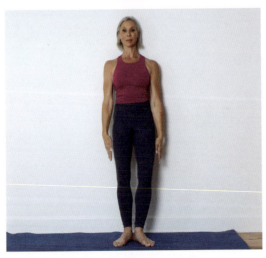

Arm Circle

Follow the same setup and steps as **ARM LOWER AND LIFT FRONT,** but in Step 2 **open your arms to the sides** as you lower them back down instead of to the front.

SETUP

Stand with your back against the wall, your heels together and the balls of your feet slightly apart. Soften your knees and pull your stomach up and in. Place your arms by your sides.

STEPS

1 Inhale and **LIFT YOUR ARMS OVERHEAD** toward the ceiling, palms facing forward.

2 Exhale, **SQUEEZING ALL THE AIR OUT OF YOUR LUNGS WHILE OPENING YOUR ARMS TO THE SIDES** and then lowering them back down. That's 1 rep. Continue for the prescribed number of reps.

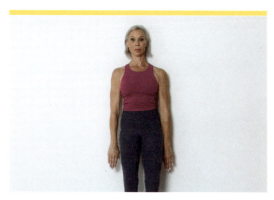

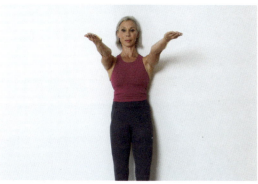

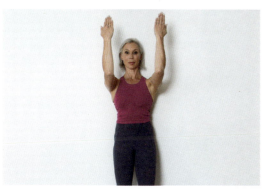

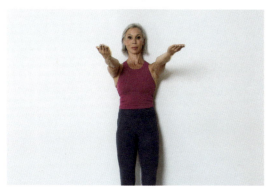

Arm Curl

SETUP

Stand with your back against the wall, your heels together and the balls of your feet slightly apart. Soften your knees and pull your stomach up and in. Place your arms by your sides.

STEPS

1 Inhale and **LIFT YOUR ARMS** to shoulder height. Exhale and rotate your palms to face the ceiling.

2 Inhale and **BEND YOUR ELBOWS LIKE YOU'RE DOING BICEPS CURLS.** Move slowly, using all your strength, as if you're holding 100 pounds in each hand. **EXTEND YOUR ARMS BACK OUT, KEEPING YOUR WRISTS STRAIGHT.** Do this 5 times, ending with your arms bent. That's 1 rep. Continue for the prescribed number of reps.

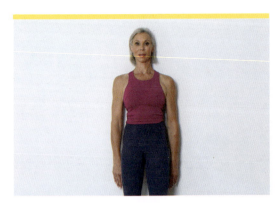

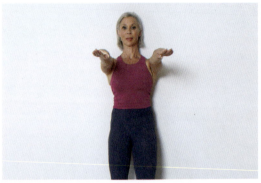

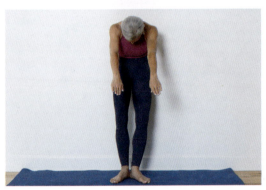

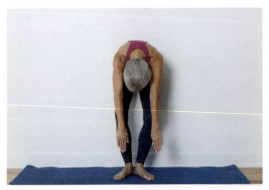

Simple Roll-Down

SETUP

Stand with your back against the wall, your heels together and the balls of your feet slightly apart. Soften your knees and pull your stomach up and in. Place your arms by your sides.

STEPS

1 Inhale and **LIFT YOUR ARMS** to shoulder height with your palms facing down. Lower your chin toward your chest.

2 Exhale and **ROUND FORWARD, PEELING YOUR UPPER BACK FROM THE WALL** while squeezing all the air out of your lungs. Let your arms dangle from your shoulders and bend your knees slightly.

3 Inhale and return to upright, **ROLLING YOUR SPINE ALONG THE WALL.** Continue letting your arms hang. That's 1 rep. Continue for the prescribed number of reps.

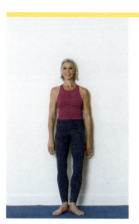
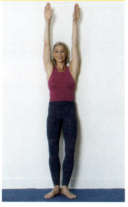
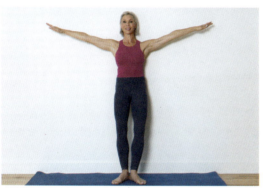
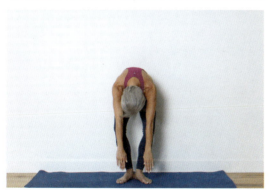

Roll-Down With Arm Circle

SETUP

Stand with your back leaning against the wall, heels together and about 6 inches from the wall. The balls of your feet should be one hand's-width apart. Soften your knees, lengthen your spine, and place your arms by your sides.

STEPS

1 Inhale deeply and **LIFT YOUR ARMS OVERHEAD** with palms facing forward.

2 Exhale, squeezing all the air out of the lungs as you **LOWER YOUR ARMS TO YOUR SIDES AND FOLD FORWARD** from the waist, tucking your chin into your chest.

3 Inhale, lift your arms forward, and roll your torso up the wall from your waist. **BRING YOUR ARMS OVERHEAD AS THE BACK OF YOUR HEAD RETURNS TO TOUCH THE WALL.** That's 1 rep. Continue for the prescribed number of reps; then repeat, reversing the movement so you start bent over and lift your arms to the sides as you roll up.

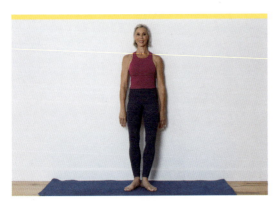

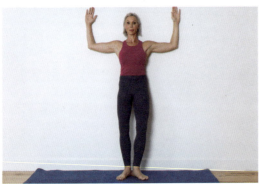

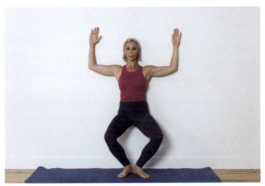

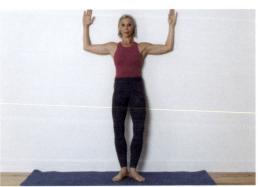

Bend and Extend Knees

SETUP

Stand with your back against the wall, heels together and balls of your feet slightly apart. Soften your knees and pull your stomach up and in. Place your arms by your sides.

STEPS

1 Inhale and **LIFT YOUR ARMS TO SHOULDER HEIGHT.**

2 Exhale and **BEND YOUR ELBOWS TO MAKE 90-DEGREE ANGLES** while raising your arms parallel to the wall, like a goalpost. Keep your entire arm pressed against the wall

3 **BEND YOUR KNEES AND SLIDE YOUR BACK DOWN THE WALL**, keeping your knees over your second toe. Straighten your knees and slide back up the wall. That's 1 rep. Continue for the prescribed number of reps.

CHALLENGE

For a greater challenge, try this move, **HANDS ROTATE DOWN AND UP,** and **BEND AND EXTEND KNEES WITH SHAVE** while holding a 1- or 2-pound weight in each hand (or use soup cans).

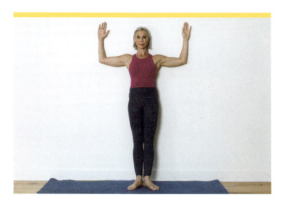

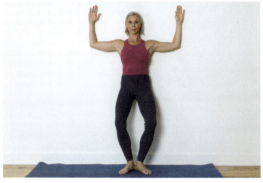

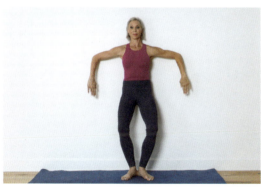

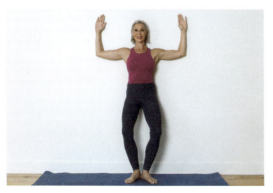

Hands Rotate Down and Up

Follow the same setup and steps as **BEND AND EXTEND KNEES,** but after bending your knees in Step 3 **rotate your arms to lower your hands forward and then down,** so your palms reach toward the wall, then reverse the motion.

SETUP

Stand with your back against the wall, your heels together and the balls of your feet slightly apart. Soften your knees and pull your stomach up and in. Place your arms by your sides.

STEPS

1 Inhale and **LIFT YOUR ARMS** to shoulder height.

2 Exhale and **BEND YOUR ELBOWS TO MAKE 90-DEGREE ANGLES** while raising your arms parallel to the wall, like a goalpost.

3 **BEND YOUR KNEES AND SLIDE** your back down the wall.

4 Rotate your arms to **LOWER YOUR HANDS FORWARD AND THEN DOWN,** so your palms reach toward the wall.

5 **LIFT YOUR HANDS FORWARD AND THEN UP, PRESSING YOUR ELBOWS AND THE BACKS OF YOUR HANDS AGAINST THE WALL.** Straighten your knees and slide back up the wall. That's 1 rep. Continue for the prescribed number of reps.

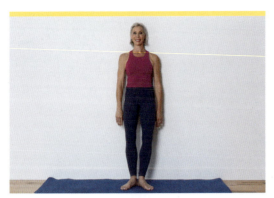

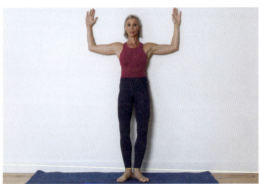

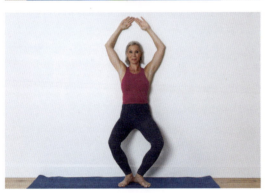

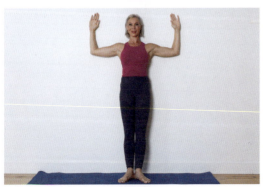

Bend and Extend Knees With Shave

Follow the same setup and steps as
BEND AND EXTEND KNEES,
but after bending your knees in Step 3
**slide your hands toward each other
to form a diamond overhead.**
Return your arms to the goalpost position
as you straighten your knees.

SETUP

Stand with your back against the wall, heels together and balls of your feet slightly apart. Soften your knees and pull your stomach up and in. Place your arms by your sides.

STEPS

1 Inhale and **LIFT YOUR ARMS** to shoulder height.

2 Exhale and **BEND YOUR ELBOWS TO MAKE 90-DEGREE ANGLES** while raising your arms parallel to the wall, like a goalpost.

3 Bend your knees and slide your back down the wall. As your knees bend, **SLIDE YOUR HANDS TOWARD EACH OTHER TO FORM A DIAMOND OVERHEAD.**

4 Straighten your knees and slide back up the wall. As your knees straighten, **SLIDE YOUR HANDS BACK DOWN TO THE GOALPOST POSITION.** That's 1 rep. Continue for the prescribed number of reps.

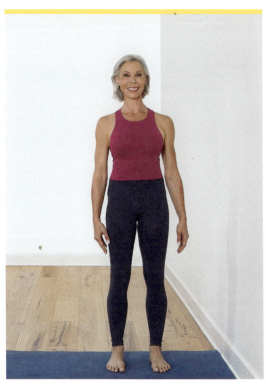

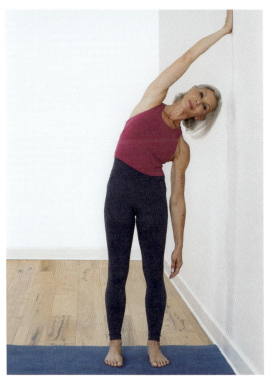

Side Bend 1

CHECK YOUR FORM

AVOID LOCKING your joints
and keep your hips and shoulders in alignment

AVOID TWISTING your legs,
hips, or shoulders

SETUP

Stand with your left side to the wall, arms at your sides and feet slightly past hip-width apart.

STEPS

1 **LIFT YOUR RIGHT ARM UP AND BEND TO THE LEFT** to reach to the wall.

2 Reverse the action and **LIFT YOUR PALM OFF THE WALL AS YOU RETURN UPRIGHT.** That's 1 rep. Continue for the prescribed number of reps; repeat on the other side.

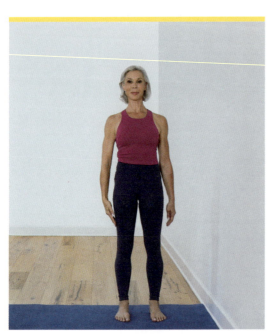

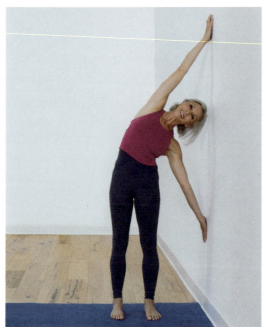

Side Bend 2

SETUP

Stand with your left side to the wall, arms at your sides and feet slightly past hip-width apart.

STEPS

1 **LIFT YOUR RIGHT ARM UP AND BEND TO THE LEFT** to reach to the wall; while reaching, bring your left palm to the wall.

2 Reverse the action and **LIFT YOUR PALM OFF THE WALL AS YOU RETURN UPRIGHT.** That's 1 rep. Continue for the prescribed number of reps; repeat on the other side.

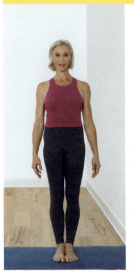
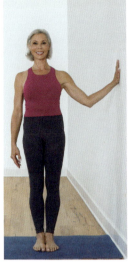
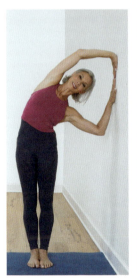
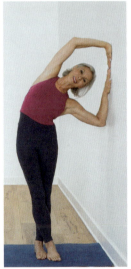

Side Bend 3

SETUP

Stand with your left side very close to the wall and your legs together. Bend your left elbow and press your hand to the wall, fingertips pointing up.

STEPS

1 Lift your right arm up and reach the wall, increasing the bend in your left arm as you reach. **PLACE YOUR RIGHT PALM ON THE WALL WITH YOUR RIGHT AND LEFT FINGERTIPS POINTING TOWARD EACH OTHER.** (The top hand may remain with fingertips toward the ceiling if pointing your fingers down is too difficult.)

2 Cross your right leg in front of your left leg. **PRESS INTO YOUR HANDS AND LEAN INTO YOUR RIGHT HIP,** stretching your right side.

3 Uncross your legs. Reverse the action, **LIFTING YOUR RIGHT PALM OFF OF THE WALL TO RETURN TO YOUR STARTING POSITION.** That's 1 rep. Continue for the prescribed number of reps; repeat on the other side.

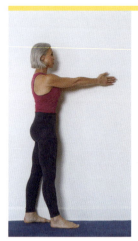
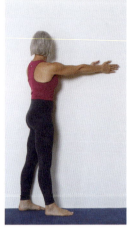
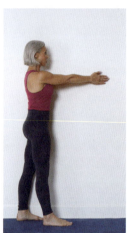
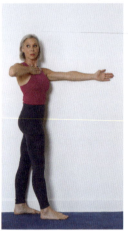
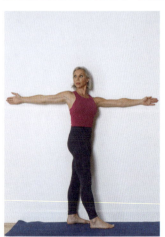
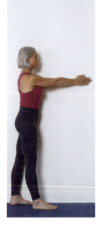

Book Covers

CHECK YOUR FORM

AVOID LOCKING your joints and keep your hips and shoulders in alignment

AVOID TWISTING your legs, hips, or shoulders

SETUP

Stand with your left side close to the wall with your right leg front, left leg back, and toes pointing forward.

STEPS

1 Extend your arms forward along the wall to shoulder height. While gazing to the wall, **REACH YOUR RIGHT PALM TO YOUR LEFT PALM.**

2 **SLIDE YOUR RIGHT HAND FORWARD PAST YOUR LEFT HAND,** then return it back to your left hand.

3 Bend your right elbow and **SLIDE YOUR RIGHT HAND ALONG YOUR LEFT ARM AND ACROSS YOUR CHEST TO EXTEND YOUR RIGHT ARM STRAIGHT OPEN DIRECTLY TO YOUR SIDE.** Continue twisting until the back of your right hand presses on the wall. Your gaze should follow your hand.

4 Reverse the rotation with your right arm extended. **RETURN YOUR RIGHT PALM TO YOUR LEFT PALM.** That's 1 rep. Continue for the prescribed number of reps; repeat on the other side.

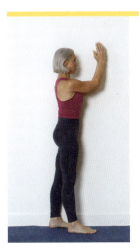
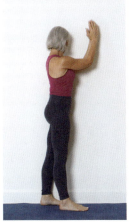
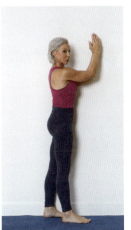
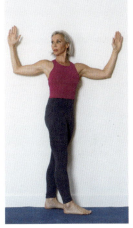
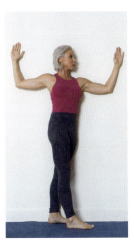
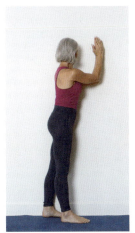

Prayer

CHECK YOUR FORM

AVOID LOCKING your joints and keep your hips and shoulders in alignment

AVOID TWISTING your legs, hips, or shoulders

SETUP

Stand with your left side close to the wall with your right leg front, left leg back, and toes pointing forward. Bend your left arm up along the wall with your elbow at shoulder height.

STEPS

1 **TOUCH YOUR RIGHT PALM TO YOUR LEFT PALM. TOUCH YOUR CHIN TO YOUR LEFT SHOULDER.**

2 **ROTATE YOUR CHIN** to touch your right shoulder.

3 Open your right arm to the side and **ROTATE TOWARD YOUR RIGHT.**

4 **ROTATE YOUR CHIN TOWARD YOUR LEFT SHOULDER.**

5 Reverse the rotation with your right arm at shoulder level. **RETURN YOUR RIGHT HAND TO YOUR LEFT PALM.**
That's 1 rep. Continue for the prescribed number of reps; repeat on the other side.

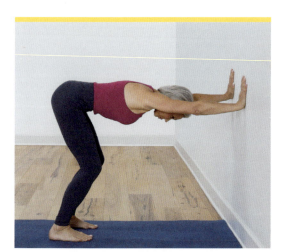

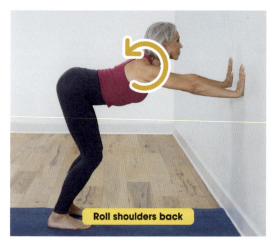

Roll shoulders back

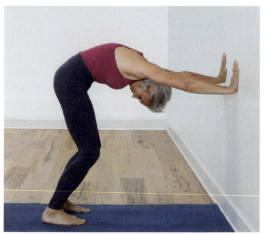

Cat and Cow With Bent Knees

CHECK YOUR FORM

AVOID LOCKING your joints and keep your hips and shoulders in alignment

KEEP your neck long

SETUP

Stand with your hands against the wall at shoulder height. Walk your feet back until your torso is flat like a tabletop. Keep your legs hip-width apart.

STEPS

1 **INHALE WHILE PRESSING YOUR HANDS** to the wall and bending your knees.

2 Roll your shoulders to your ears and circle them back and down to lift your head. As your head lifts, **EXHALE AND ARCH YOUR ENTIRE SPINE, LIFTING YOUR CHEST FORWARD.** Inhale and return to tabletop position.

3 **EXHALE AND ROUND FORWARD, ARCHING YOUR SPINE LIKE A SCARED CAT.** Inhale and return to tabletop position. That's 1 rep. Continue for the prescribed number of reps.

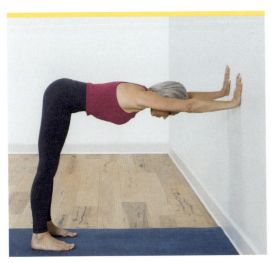

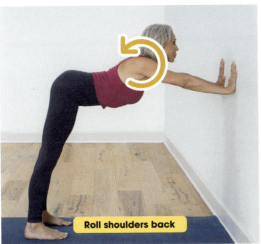

Roll shoulders back

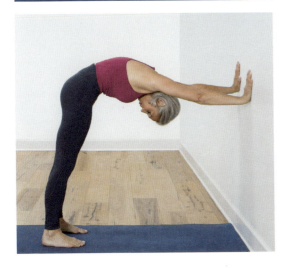

Cat and Cow With Straight Knees

Follow the same setup and steps as **CAT AND COW WITH BENT KNEES,** but in Step 1 **keep your legs straight instead of bending them.**

SETUP

Stand with your hands against the wall at shoulder height. Walk your feet back until your torso is flat like a tabletop. Keep your legs hips-width apart.

STEPS

1 Inhale and press your hands to the wall, **KEEPING YOUR LEGS STRAIGHT BUT NOT LOCKED.**

2 Roll your shoulders to your ears and circle them back and down to lift your head. As your head lifts, **EXHALE AND ARCH YOUR ENTIRE SPINE, LIFTING YOUR CHEST FORWARD.** Inhale and return to tabletop position.

3 **EXHALE AND ROUND FORWARD, ARCHING YOUR SPINE LIKE A SCARED CAT.** Inhale and return to tabletop position. That's 1 rep. Continue for the prescribed number of reps.

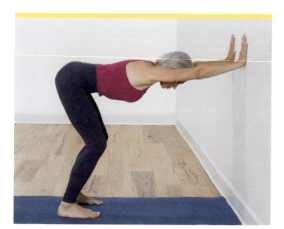

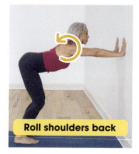

Roll shoulders back

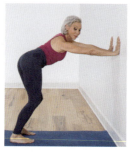

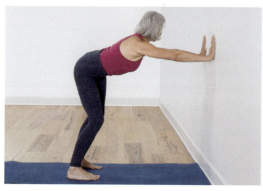

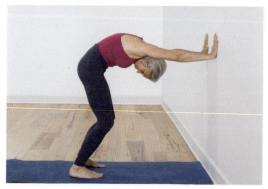

Curious Cat and Cow With Bent Knees

Follow the same setup and steps as **CAT AND COW WITH BENT KNEES,** but after Step 3 **inhale and turn your head to the right while bending your tailbone to the right.** Exhale and return to center. Repeat to the left.

SETUP

Stand with your hands against the wall at shoulder height. Walk your feet back until your torso is flat like a tabletop. Keep your legs hip-width apart.

STEPS

1 **INHALE WHILE PRESSING YOUR HANDS** to the wall and bending your knees.

2 Roll your shoulders to your ears and circle them back and down to lift your head. As your head lifts, **EXHALE AND ARCH YOUR ENTIRE SPINE, LIFTING YOUR CHEST FORWARD.** Inhale and return to tabletop position.

3 Inhale and **TURN YOUR HEAD TO THE RIGHT WHILE BENDING YOUR TAILBONE TO THE RIGHT.** Exhale and return to center. Repeat to the left.

4 Inhale deeply. **EXHALE AND ROUND FORWARD, ARCHING YOUR SPINE LIKE A SCARED CAT.** Inhale and return to tabletop position. That's 1 rep. Continue for the prescribed number of reps.

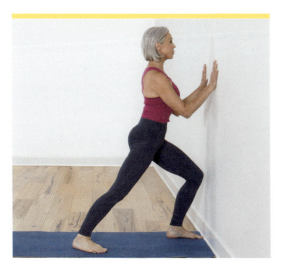

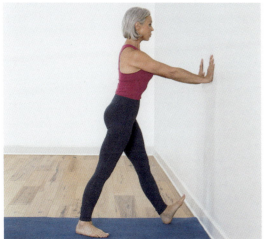

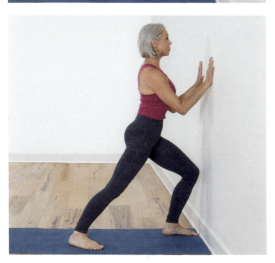

Extend and Bend

CHECK YOUR FORM

AVOID LOCKING your joints and keep your hips and shoulders in alignment

SETUP

Stand with your hands against the wall at shoulder height with elbows bent down. Lunge your left leg forward, bending it at a 90-degree angle. Keep your right leg straight with your foot turned out 45 degrees.

STEPS

1 Press your hips back to straighten your left leg and arms. **FLEX YOUR LEFT FOOT.** Lower your toes and re-bend your left leg.

2 **LIFT YOUR CHEST, SQUEEZING YOUR SHOULDER BLADES TOGETHER.**
That's 1 rep. Continue for the prescribed number of reps.

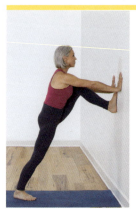
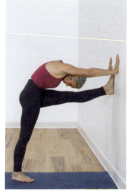
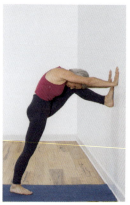
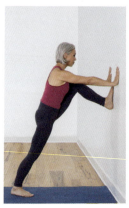

Extend and Bend: Foot on Wall

SETUP

Stand facing the wall. Place your left foot on the wall with your knee bent, toes and knee pointing toward the ceiling. Place your hands on the wall with your arms straight at shoulder height. Keep your right leg straight with your foot turned out 45 degrees.

STEPS

1 **EXTEND YOUR LEFT LEG WHILE ROUNDING YOUR BACK** to bring your forehead toward your knee.

2 **BEND YOUR LEFT KNEE.** Keep your arms straight but not locked.

3 **LIFT YOUR CHEST AND SQUEEZE YOUR SHOULDER BLADES TOGETHER.** That's 1 rep. Continue for the prescribed number of reps.

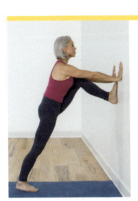
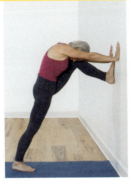
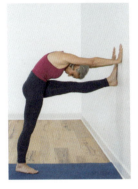
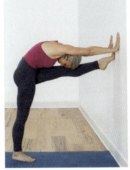
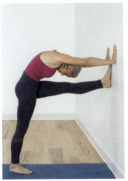
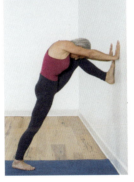
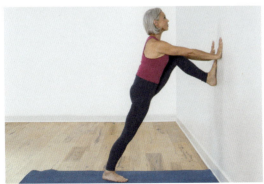

Extend and Bend: Foot on Wall With Heel Lift

Follow the same setup and steps as
EXTEND AND BEND: FOOT ON WALL
but after Step 1 **lift and lower
your right heel.**

SETUP

Stand facing the wall. Place your left foot on the wall with your knee bent, toes and knee pointing toward the ceiling. Place your hands on the wall with your arms straight at shoulder height. Keep your right leg straight with your foot turned out 45 degrees.

STEPS

1 **EXTEND YOUR LEFT LEG WHILE ROUNDING YOUR BACK** to bring your forehead toward your knee.

2 **LIFT YOUR LEFT HEEL. LOWER YOUR LEFT HEEL.**

3 **BEND YOUR LEFT KNEE.** Keep your arms straight but not locked.

4 **LIFT YOUR CHEST AND SQUEEZE YOUR SHOULDER BLADES TOGETHER.** That's 1 rep. Continue for the prescribed number of reps.

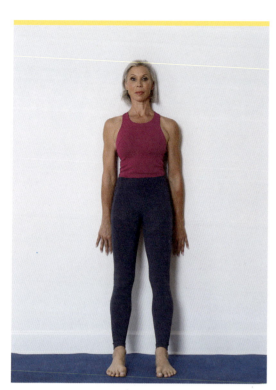

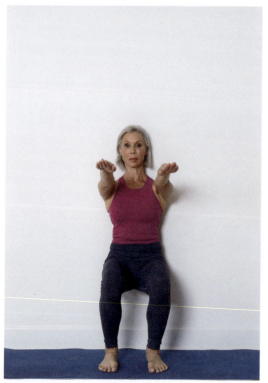

Extend and Bend Squat

SETUP

Stand with your back and arms against the wall with feet sit-bone distance apart. To find how far your feet should be from the wall to perform your squat, bend your knees and slide your back down the wall. Walk your feet forward until you create a 90-degree angle. Straighten your knees.

STEPS

1 Inhale deeply. **EXHALE AND LIFT YOUR ARMS TO SHOULDER HEIGHT WHILE BENDING YOUR LEGS INTO A SQUAT.** Hold for 3 to 5 seconds.

2 **STRAIGHTEN YOUR KNEES TO LENGTHEN YOUR SPINE ALONG THE WALL.** Lower your arms. That's 1 rep. Continue for the prescribed number of reps.

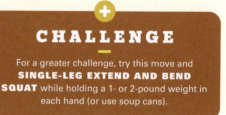

+ CHALLENGE

For a greater challenge, try this move and **SINGLE-LEG EXTEND AND BEND SQUAT** while holding a 1- or 2-pound weight in each hand (or use soup cans).

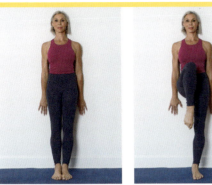

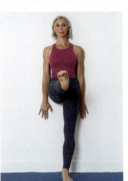
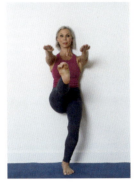

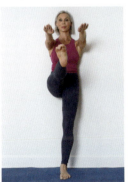
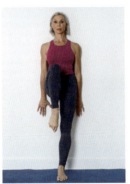

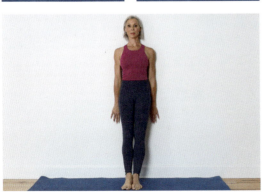

Single-Leg Extend and Bend Squat

SETUP

Stand with your back and arms against the wall with feet together. To find how far your feet should be from the wall to perform your squat, bend your knees and slide your back down the wall. Walk your feet forward until you create a 90-degree angle. Straighten your knees.

STEPS

1 Inhale deeply, **BENDING YOUR RIGHT LEG TOWARD YOUR CHEST THEN EXTENDING IT FORWARD.** (You can keep your knee bent if needed.)

2 Exhale and **LIFT YOUR ARMS TO SHOULDER HEIGHT AND BEND YOUR LEFT LEG INTO A SQUAT.** Hold for 3 to 5 seconds.

3 **STRAIGHTEN YOUR LEFT LEG TO LENGTHEN YOUR SPINE ALONG THE WALL.**

4 **BEND YOUR RIGHT KNEE TO YOUR CHEST AND PLACE YOUR FOOT BACK ON THE FLOOR.** Lower you arms. That's 1 rep. Continue for the prescribed number of reps.

Prevention is a registered trademark of Hearst Magazines, Inc.

Book design by Kevin Su

Library of Congress Cataloging-in-Publication Data is on file with the publisher.

ISBN 978-1-955710-33-6

Printed in China

2 4 6 8 10 9 7 5 3 1 hardcover

HEARST

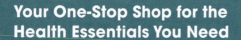